Advance Praise for *Always Eat Dessert...*

"Mary Lou's thoughts on dining in restaurants are spot on. You don't have to throw away all of your hard work and restraint just because you are going out to eat. One can easily look at a restaurant's menu online, and if you can't find something that will not totally throw your diet into a tailspin, I would suggest calling the restaurant and speaking to the chef. Any chef worth his salt should be more than willing to accommodate any dietary needs you have. We do it for people with gluten sensitivity and allergies, so why not for those wanting to watch calories? Also, good restaurants always have light and healthy options available."

—Bill Rodgers, Executive Chef,
Keens Steakhouse, NYC

"The main thing here is that it is not a matter of just getting up and 'moving,' which is at least a start as Mary Lou mentions in her chapter 'Being a Couch Potato Is Okay,' but it is focusing and actually exerting yourself. People who start to exercise on a regular basis usually do not lose weight but change their body make-up. They start to look slimmer. One of the benefits of a regular exercise program is that over time your body will start to change its cravings for more healthy combinations of foods. An additional benefit of a regular exercise routine is that it gives you time to focus mentally on other things, which will help lower your stress levels. This is a connection Mary Lou makes throughout her book in several ways. Many of the people that trained with us lowered their need for diabetic medicine, blood pressure medicine, and stress medication. So go ahead and give it a shot; the only thing you have to lose is some weight."

—Bert Johnson and Jeanne Vlazny,
Marathon Training Coaches

"As a fashion stylist, I find this book easy to read and compelling. Mary Lou's knowledge on fashion and what works for losing weight, keeping it off, and looking your best NOW are all helpful tools. As Mary Lou says, 'Wear the right clothes to look good now.' You will feel great on the inside because you look fabulous on the outside."

—Candy DeLapp,
Independent Fashion Consultant

"Stand or sit up straight!...The phrase, 'I am' becomes strong in the power of Mary Lou's words in the chapter entitled, 'Always Take Time for Yourself.' Mary Lou invites us to love ourselves so that we can love others. We can do this by being mindful in the present moment. Mindfulness is something I practice myself. I encourage those whom I counsel to do this also. I enjoyed the chapter 'Always Take Time for Yourself' and found it helpful for my own life."

—Sister Mary Jean Ferry,
BVM, Spiritual Director

ALWAYS EAT DESSERT

and 6 More Weight Loss and Lifestyle Habits I Learned in the Convent

MARY LOU REID

Post Hill
PRESS

A POST HILL PRESS BOOK

ISBN: 978-1-68261-667-3
ISBN (eBook): 978-1-68261-668-0

Always Eat Dessert…
and 6 More Weight Loss Lifestyle Habits I Learned in the Convent
© 2018 by Mary Lou Reid
All Rights Reserved

Cover art by Dan Pitts

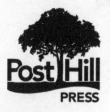

Post Hill Press
New York • Nashville
posthillpress.com

Published in the United States of America

This book is dedicated to all those who have ever dieted...dieted...dieted...and given up.

Contents

Part IV. Upon Reflection...What I Have Learned

References

T his is the book you need to read after you have lost weight, and you need to refer to it for the rest of your life.

Did you buy this book because you have lost and regained the same 20, 30, 40, or 50 pounds *again and again…and again*?

May Lou Reid has maintained her weight loss for 50 years, and she shares how she has done it. As you know, if you have lost weight and gained it back, you need to know what to do in order to maintain your new weight. If you go back to the behaviors that caused you to gain weight, the weight will come back!

Along with the techniques and strategies she has used to successfully keep the weight off, she shares delightful stories about life as a nun, and reflections 50 years later when she takes a trip back to the convent. This book is a delightful blend of diet advice with a little philosophy thrown in.

This book fills a void. There are hundreds, probably thousands, of books that tell you how to lose weight; this book gives you effective ways to *keep it off!*

As a registered dietitian, I have spoken to so many people (men and women of all ages) over the past 19 years who have said: "I lost weight [on whatever diet], but then it all came back…and then some." In *Always Eat Dessert*, the author shares how she avoided gaining weight back and how you can too.

Some people do well with the structure of a diet: they don't have to think about it; they just follow it, whether it's restricting calories, fat, or carbs, or buying prepared meals. But once the weight has been lost, and the structure is gone, it's easy to slide back into old patterns of behavior that gradually lead to weight gain.

This is the book you need to read when your diet ends. That's when it's time to take it to another level, the "I never want to see those pounds again" level.

As Mary Lou says, this is not a quick weight-loss diet; it's a lifestyle change.

This book is filled with useful advice about how to maintain your weight loss from someone who has actually been successful at it for 50 years.

What I love about this book is that Mary Lou tells you that this is an ongoing struggle, and shares her own experiences with that struggle.

Most people don't lose weight and magically keep it off; it takes consistent effort. I love when she talks about going back to the convent after many years, and how things have changed. Instead of meals being served, they are now buffet style. Mary Lou talks about gaining a few pounds while she was there, and how she got back on track (using her course correction and quick tips).

It's not always possible to focus on your diet the way you do when you are losing weight. Life happens; there are vacations, family gatherings, celebrations, stress, and other things that cause your weight to fluctuate, but the key is to correct your course and lose extra pounds before it goes too far. Mary Lou shares her strategies to compensate for pounds that start to come back on. You can certainly lose weight on a diet, but you need to develop habits that will help you maintain your weight for a lifetime.

She shares excellent tips you can use while eating in restaurants, and what she does to satisfy cravings without overindulging. Deprivation diets work for a short time, but you *can* incorporate the foods you love back into your life. After the weight-loss diet ends, you can enjoy the foods you love again; you shouldn't put an end to the joy of eating.

Behaviors that lead to weight creeping back on: eating out frequently, a decrease in exercise, celebrations, holidays, and other things that cause a change in your daily routine.

Everyone is different. It's important to find out what works for you, and continue doing it. We all get off track, but the key is to know that this is going to happen and to go back to the things that work for you.

Her reflections on life in the convent, and her observations after returning 50 years later, are fascinating. It was interesting to peek into a world I knew nothing about.

Mary Lou talks about portion control rather than calorie counting. She talks about how she lost weight, and how she maintains her weight by eating dessert daily; it can be done.

This book is Mary Lou's story, and as I said before, everyone is different and what works for one person may not work for you, but I know you will find many strategies that will help you maintain your weight. Many of them are recommendations I make to my clients and patients, and follow myself.

You can use this book as your weight maintenance guide for the rest of your life!

— Joyce Berenson, RD, CDE, is a Registered Dietitian Nutritionist and a Certified Diabetes Educator in Temecula, California. For more information, please visit www.diabetesdiet4life.com.

Foreword II

I am a clinical psychologist who specializes in obsessive-compulsive disorder and has worked in the eating disorder field for more than ten years. I have been in practice over 40 years. I do evaluations for people requesting bariatric surgery, and I run a support group for people who have completed bariatric surgery. I believe that this book espouses extremely valid principles and ways that one can lose weight and keep it off. What Mary Lou Reid states is nothing new but the way she states it and how she puts it together make extremely good clinical sense. The psychological principles are sound. Breaking a habit is extremely difficult. If you follow the tenets put forth in this book, it is highly likely that you can lose weight and, if you follow through with the principles, keep it off. The basic principles that work here are persistence and consistency. When the author recalls her time in the convent, you can see that this is exactly the type of behavior that led her to be able to lose 50 pounds and keep it off for 50 years. Working with weight loss is more difficult than most any other obsessive behavior. If people smoke or drink and want to stop, they can quit. With weight, you have to learn to moderate, and that is central to Mary Lou's advice. If you are able to follow what the author is saying and be persistent in your continued attempt to modify your eating behaviors, it is likely that you will be successful in losing weight and keeping it off. It has to be a lifestyle change. Don't forget the title, however: *Always Eat Dessert*.

Richard S. Klein, Ph.D.
Richard S. Klein, Ph.D. is a licensed psychologist who has been practicing in the Los Angeles area for 40 years and has a specialty in treating obsessive-compulsive disorders which often relate to weight problems and over-eating.

Introduction

L osing weight is usually the number-one New Year's resolution for men and women of all ages. More than 35 percent of our country today is statistically considered obese, and another 40 percent is overweight. There are many weight-loss books and plans on the market, but most cannot effectively help people keep the weight off for a lifetime. *Always Eat Dessert...and 6 More Weight Loss and Lifestyle Habits I Learned in the Convent* can do that.

Mine is the story of accidental weight loss. I never thought about losing weight when I entered the convent, but it happened. The eating habits I learned in the convent stayed with me for a lifetime.

In 1965, I entered the convent. I was a young girl, just out of high school, who was very idealistic and wanted to live the perfect life. My vision was to dedicate my life to God by helping others. I also happened to be about 50 pounds overweight. Perhaps I felt that the convent was the perfect place to be accepted by others for myself and not for what I looked like. Thus began my unexpected weight-loss journey. I lost 50 pounds and kept the weight off for 50 years. I tell my story of accidental weight loss through real stories of convent life as it was 50 years ago, and as I lived it in the convent through 1970, highlighting the habits I learned then, in what I affectionately refer to as the Convent Diet. I explain why those habits work today and how to turn them into lifetime habits. I have friends who entered the convent with me those many years ago who also have maintained the significant weight loss they achieved then.

I am writing this book because my story can be someone else's new beginning, someone else's path to permanent weight loss. Be assured: losing weight the convent way does not require entering a convent!

This book is for anyone who:

- Wants to lose weight "the accidental way" and keep it off for a lifetime
- Has tried everything else and failed to lose weight and keep it off
- Has lost weight with great effort and sacrifice but is struggling to keep it off forever
- Wants to "get a life" and put weight loss on the back burner

This is *my* story. There are many other convents and periods of time in convent life that may have been different from what I experienced. Others in my group who shared my same experiences may have seen those experiences differently and therefore experienced a different convent life from mine. There were also young girls in my group who gained a bit of weight (too much delicious homemade bread) or neither gained nor lost weight. That I and others lost weight and kept it off for a lifetime remains remarkable.

Life in the convent prepared me to write this book not only because I lost 50 pounds and kept it off for 50 years, but also because I learned other life-changing habits and core values that allowed me to continue living my ideal life of helping others, tempered with reality—getting through two breast surgeries—and bolstered by the confidence needed to survive in the world. The formation, as the convent instruction was called, stuck with me for 50 years and guided me through a brief career in the arts in New York and on to a 30-plus-year career as a financial planner. The work of a Certified Financial Planner is certainly that of helping and guiding others, which is what I sought to do in the convent.

Many people have searched for the secret to permanent weight loss. Many people have a great curiosity about the secrets of convent life, especially convent life as it was in the days before and during the great changes that took place in the Catholic Church beginning with Vatican II and Pope John XXIII in the 1960s. I am in the unique position of having maintained a significant weight loss over a long lifetime as well as having lived as a nun in the convent of yesterday.

My book is about an 18-year-old heavyset girl without a whole lot of self-confidence and with a houseful of younger brothers. This young woman enters a convent planning to stay forever, living an idealistic life devoted to God. Perhaps deep down she is also looking for peer acceptance while fighting the parental disapproval of her decision. She leaves the convent a lot lighter, and those pounds never come back.

The young woman practices time-tested weight management principles without even realizing it, because it is just part of the rule of convent life. She sits down for dinner and is served a predetermined portion of a predetermined food. The only thing that keeps her from leaving the table ravenously hungry is *dessert*.

The Convent Diet isn't really a diet at all. It is a way of looking at food and dealing with life. It is a way of making food your friend instead of your enemy. It is a way of thinking positively about food, because negative diets full of "don'ts" and "shouldn'ts" can't last a lifetime.

The Convent Diet is a guide to creating your own personal diet, inspired, perhaps, by reading what worked for me. The key to losing weight and keeping it off is an individual thing. For most people, it *does* take trial and error.

Trendy diets may all work in the short term. Trendy diets generally don't work in the long term.

The Convent Diet is neither a trendy diet nor a magic-bullet diet. Yes, I eat dessert every day, and yes, I consider myself a couch potato because I spend most of each day seated in an office swivel chair or on the couch reading and watching TV. However, there are *three musts* for success with the Convent Diet:

- The determination to create good habits, and to create and practice a routine
- The tenacity to stick with it and start again, as many times as is necessary
- The ability to face "the elephant in the room" created by the times we live in: *stress*

I'm going to address these three musts as I discuss the Seven Holy Habits, by sharing convent and personal experiences and successes of my own on each of these three topics.

The book is laid out as follows:

FOREWORDS

Forewords from both a registered dietitian and a psychologist who believe the habits discussed in this book make sense

MY JOURNEY TO THE CONVENT DIET

Short stories or "vignettes," called "A Midcentury Slice of Convent Life."

GETTING INTO THE HABITS

The three musts, plus tips for accomplishing all three over the long term:
- Create habits
- Stick to the habits
- Handle stress

THE SEVEN HOLY HABITS

- Visualization: You're thin until you're thin
- Always eat dessert
- Don't count calories, but calories count
- Being a couch potato is okay
- Don't be on a diet in a restaurant
- Opt out of fake food
- Always take time for yourself

UPON REFLECTION...WHAT I HAVE LEARNED: A COLLECTION OF CONVENT REFLECTIONS

These reflections generally start with the observation of the smallest, simplest thing—a bird, a squirrel, a cloud—and expand into contemplation of a core life value, which is generally brought home with a weight-loss insight. The home chef will enjoy the historical recipes from the *Kitchen of Tomorrow* radio broadcasts of over 50 years ago.

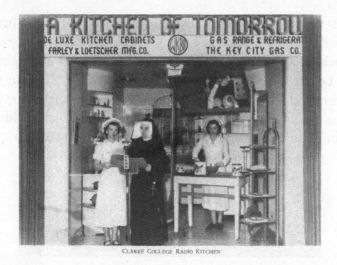

CLARKE COLLEGE RADIO KITCHEN

Kitchen of Tomorrow Radio Broadcast set of the 1940s, program moderated by Sister St. Clara, home economist and chairman of the home economics department, Clarke College, Dubuque, Iowa

REFERENCE SECTION

This section of the book is a quick reference section. Each topic can work as a quick action tool, whether you read the book cover to cover or not. There are quick tips for the long term, a daily accountability checker, course correction ideas, and a glossary of convent terminology.

AFTERWORD—A CALL TO ACTION, TITLED "MARCH ON"

This book can be read through start to finish or it can be used as a reference book, with points used as needed.

This book can also be paired with almost any other weight-loss system to be used as a lifelong weight-maintenance plan once the weight has been lost.

Always Eat Dessert is a lifestyle book. Anyone who has tried to lose weight and gained it back will relish this book. Anyone looking for a lifestyle change will be inspired by the reflections and stories from the convent. Those wanting to reach back and relish the delightful charm of a simpler time will read this book and enjoy the convent vignettes and pictures.

Losing weight is an individual process. You should do what is best based on your individual needs and wishes. For many, seeking the guidance of a professional such as a dietitian or psychologist is step one. For others, professional consultation may be desired along with other self-help steps, or not at all. I am neither an expert nor a professional in the area of weight loss, but I certainly believe in using professional help and advice. I am simply telling my own story and relating what has worked for me throughout my lifetime.

And for me, following the habits of the Convent Diet banishes forever the need for that number-one New Year's resolution: lose weight.

PART I

MY JOURNEY TO DISCOVER THE CONVENT DIET

A Midcentury Slice of Convent Life

I n my discussions with people about the Convent Diet, I have learned that often there is as much interest in convent life, especially in convent life as it was more than 50 years ago, as there is in the diet principles themselves.

Part I shares a few stories or vignettes from convent life as I recall them personally and as they have been told to me by nun friends. This book is not a personal memoir, though I use personal convent experiences throughout the book to illustrate weight-loss issues and principles.

I begin my story with a day in the life of a nun as I lived it. These stories illustrate my Seven Holy Habits, and I note when each is explained for the first time.

ENTRANCE DAY AND A DAY IN THE LIFE OF A NOVICE

On July 31, 1965, my mother drove me to the Union Depot in St. Paul, Minnesota, to board a Chicago Great Western passenger train, complete with dome cars, to make the approximately four-hour trip to Dubuque, Iowa. Chicago Great Western had owned the route between St. Paul and Dubuque since the 1800s. The common trains running in 1965 included the Burlington Zephyr, a diesel train, combined with either the Empire Builder or the North Coast Limited. I remember all the names well.

This was my second visit to the train station. My first was an exciting adventure with my grandmother in the 1950s. She and I traveled to Chicago for the weekend and stayed in a hotel together. It was on that trip that I fell in love with Chicago, especially its Chinatown. I still have a pair of screw-back earrings I picked out in Chinatown. Don't ask me why I picked out earrings, as I was too young to wear such things. Now, Chicago was about to become a big part of my life again, as I became a nun.

I walked into the cavernous domed structure that was the depot and just looked up at the ornate ceiling and felt as though I was in a palace. The Fourth Street entrance to Union Depot is in the neoclassical style. The concourse and the waiting room that extend over the tracks are viewed as a great architectural neoclassical achievement. The building, originally built between 1917 and 1923, was added to the National Register of Historical Places in 1974.

Then I looked around at the sea of wooden benches and the variety of souls sitting, lounging, and sleeping on them. That majestic dome had feet of clay. Even 50 years ago there were what appeared to be homeless people claiming their piece of real estate in the depot. There were the "all aboard" calls for different track numbers over the loudspeaker and the general hustle and bustle of a large public business.

I really don't remember a lot of conversation with my mother while I waited. It was an awkward time. My parents were against my entering the convent, especially my father. Nor do I remember where my four brothers and father were at the time. It was a Saturday, so none were in school or at work. Other girls from my high school were also entering the convent that day, but I don't remember seeing any of them until we got off the train and landed on a bus together, headed up the hill in Dubuque to the convent.

I enjoyed meeting some of the other girls on the bus. I remember the tone of the conversation as one of smiles and laughter. I did a lot of listening and not too much talking.

As we walked up the long path and up the steps to the front door of the convent, Sister Marcia, a friend who was a year ahead of me in high school and so a year ahead of me in the novitiate, opened the door to greet us. As we reached the top of the steps, Marcia burst into tears and explained that she was very homesick—a rather ominous greeting. Though it was now past lunch time, how could anyone be hungry or think about food at this kind of a moment? I remember thinking that I did not feel homesick at all. I was up for a big adventure and was sure that a year later, when I was in Marcia's shoes, I wouldn't miss home at all. That turned out to be true.

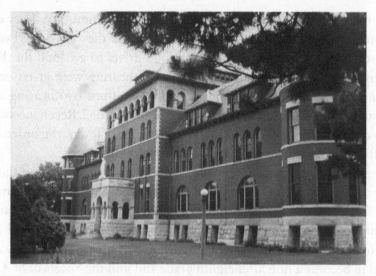

Convent I entered in the Midwest in 1965

The interior of the convent with its well-appointed sitting rooms felt elegant and formal. Little did I know at the time that I would hardly ever visit this part of the house again, as it was reserved for professed sisters and guests. At one point, I had a duty that involved buffing the wood floors, including those on the professed side of the house. That was kind of a rock 'n' roll job, as the boards would buckle in the Midwest humidity. Keeping control of the heavy buffing machine back and forth over the bumpy floor was no easy feat. I was also distracted by the beauty of the large clock whose weights and chains reached between floors.

Back to our arrival. Marcia showed us to our quarters. I don't remember whether we changed into our postulant habits immediately or the next day. I don't remember what we had for dinner that first night. A common dinner was a scoop of chicken salad (five scoops per platter, two platters per table, and ten girls per table) and a bowl of shoestring potato fries (two bowls per table with enough for five girls per bowl). You did not want to take too many shoestring potato fries for fear of leaving none for the others. And of course, there was a plate of bread on each end of the table. The dessert was something simple, like a small bowl of canned fruit or pudding. The meals were memorable for their simplicity, sparseness and, as I recall, lack of excessive preparation. Was I on an evening picnic each night? This was portion control at its finest.

At the time, this order of nuns was not a rich community. They did not pay into, nor did they receive, Social Security as they do now. I've heard many stories of parishioners putting on food drives to get food for the nuns teaching in the parish school. Sisters hard of hearing were given only one hearing aid, because the community could not afford two hearing aids for one sister. What did they need most, a bra or a girdle? Receiving both was not an option. One or the other had to be chosen. (Today, the order is quite well off and helps other orders that are struggling.)

The spiritual readings were more inspiring than the food, and the atmosphere more romantic. This convent was not as austere as the convent in the movie *The Nun's Story*, with Audrey Hepburn, but maybe only because this convent wasn't as old as the Gothic abbey portrayed in the movie. I have to admit to having been inspired by Hepburn in that movie in 1959 as a child. I wanted to become a nun after eighth grade and join the Sisters of St. Casimir in Chicago as an aspirant, but my parents forbade it. Sister Luke, as Hepburn was called in the movie, was the daughter of a surgeon, as was I, and gave up everything to serve in the Belgian Congo. I didn't quite make it to the Belgian Congo, but I did find mission experience in Kansas City, St. Louis, and St. Paul. This order of nuns was at that time a teaching order. I received a top-notch high school education from these nuns, recognized for their generally high academic level and their drive to be at the forefront of change. They were willing to push the boundaries, and I thought, "This is for me."

In the convent, our lives were ordered for us. Many choices and decisions were out of our control. The very decision to enter the convent meant, to me, anyway, at age 17, that the rest of my life's decisions would be made for me and I wouldn't have to think about hard choices anymore. Of course, that was not a totally true assumption, nor was it a good reason for entering the convent!

In the convent our "happy life" was ordered for us. The bell for us to rise rang at 5:30 a.m. Then began the ritual of washing my face in the basin of water I had brought from the community restrooms the night before and placed on top of my four-drawer commode. There were no sinks or running water in the dorms. The same water was then used to brush my teeth. Of course, it was very important to remember to wash my face first!

Each cubicle surrounded by a white curtain was called an alcove. On my dorm room floor of eight alcoves there were two very desirable window alcoves. We rotated alcoves periodically. I was assigned a window alcove during the winter. While I loved having a window draped in dark brown wooden shutters that opened to reveal an idyllic pastoral view, it meant that the face-washing/tooth-brushing ritual required another step: chipping ice from the top of the basin water. As an aside, my parents sent me two sets of one-piece fleece pajamas complete with furry feet attached to wear during my window alcove days, which I was given permission to keep. One set was pink and one set was blue, not exactly the regulation white nightgown. It was also a good thing that I had grown up in Minnesota and was quite used to cold weather—just not so much inside the house, as was the case at Mount Carmel.

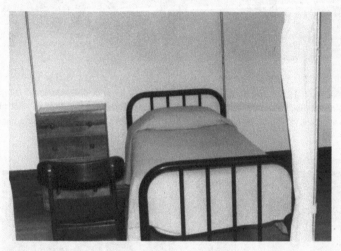

A single alcove, the width from left of dresser to right of bed, closed off for dressing by white curtain in right foreground. Basin of water brought in at night and set atop dresser for morning grooming. Each dorm room contained 8-10 alcoves and rows of rods and white curtains.

After six months as postulants, we petitioned to be received into the order. At the reception ceremony, we received the habit and the white veil of a novice.

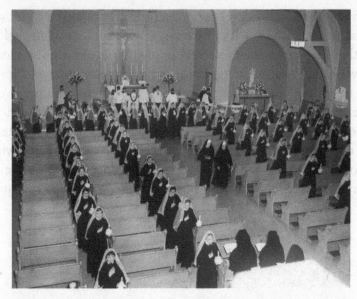

Reception, the official entrance into community, signified by reception of habit and, for many years, a "new" name, held in the Convent Chapel. Ours was the first set to be able to keep baptismal name, with a few exceptions, a recognition of Vatican II theology stressing the primacy of Baptism in the Christian vocation. My baptismal name, Mary Lou, became Sister Mary Louise, a saint's name.

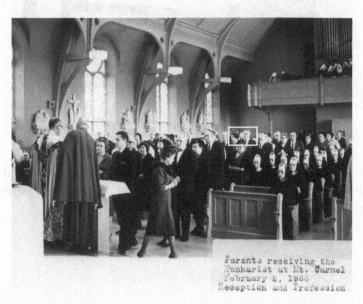

Parents' side of the chapel shown, Author's Reception day into Community, 2/2/66, with her parents marked in white box.

Then there was the march of the 55 novices in our set, plus however many more novices there were in the set ahead of me and the set behind me, to and from the toilets to dump the basin waters. Next began the getting-dressed process. Back behind my own white curtain I put on the habit: black serge pleated skirt, black cotton long-sleeved underblouse, belt, long brown wooden rosary beads, black serge cape, and white starched collar. The last step, after transitioning from a postulant to a novice, was to put on the veil. For me, that was easier said than done. The process involved covering one's head with a cap, a white, flat, starched piece that required a pleat to be made on each side of the front of the cardboard-like material. This wasn't the hardest part. Next, the veil was attached to a half-moon-shaped piece of plastic that needed to be shaped around and above the head, creating a soft point in the top middle. This shaped piece and veil required pinning on each side of the head. I would pin one side but be unable to hold the other side in place, creating a crooked point or a point too wide or too narrow. I started over with this step many times.

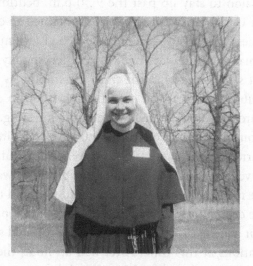
Author dressed in full habit

There was always a professed sister checking the dorms to make sure that each girl was up, dressed, and in the chapel during that half hour between 5:30 to 6:00 a.m. I was discovered one morning by the professed sister checking the dorms still in my cubicle, trying to get the pins into my headdress after 6 a.m. I was nearly in tears. I did not know the sister who discovered me, but I remember that she said nothing, seemed to smile a bit, and walked on. (I learned later from Sister Mary Teresian that smiling at humorous novice activities was frowned upon. This is a story for another chapter.) I was not reprimanded for not being in the chapel on time. I eventually made it to the chapel that morning and slipped into a pew. My tardiness was noted, I am sure, but neither recorded nor mentioned to me.

Once we were all in chapel and said a morning prayer together, it was time for a half hour of morning meditation. Though required, this was a very free and freeing time. If only I could so firmly make a half-hour meditation required in my life today! Meditation was one of my favorite times, even though I'm not a morning person and fought sleep, some mornings more than others, as you'll see.

The first year of the novitiate was called the canonical year and involved prayer, meditation, lectures in spirituality from the novice mistress, and lots of housecleaning. In the second year, we were back in school at Clarke College in Dubuque, owned and run by the sisters. I was a music major, and my classes at the college included piano lessons, requiring piano practice. I was given permission to stay up past the 9:30 p.m. bedtime to practice the piano. One of the classrooms at the novitiate contained an electric piano and a set of headphones, which I used to practice at night. I enjoyed this time to myself with the piano. While the huge convent felt spooky at night with no one around, I felt safe and cozy in the small classroom. As a "night person," I didn't have trouble staying awake even though I got up every morning at 5:30 a.m. The hard part was staying awake in the morning.

For this reason, sleeping through the 6:00 a.m. meditation was not an uncommon occurrence. For meditation, we were not required to stay in the chapel. I usually went out and walked along the pine walkway outdoors to let the fresh air wake me up. If I really couldn't hold my head up, I made a beeline to one of the classrooms, put my head down, and slept. I guess I didn't really worry about getting caught. Maybe all the professed sisters were doing their own meditations at this time. After half an hour, the bell rang, summoning us all back to the chapel for Mass. We didn't wear watches, and there was no need, as we were summoned from activity to activity by a bell system.

Mass was held in a large traditional chapel. The convent was just like one in the movies: a large red brick 1892 structure with turrets on each side, sitting on top of a hill overlooking the Mississippi River. While the chapel was only a room in the building, it was the size of a stand-alone church, with large stained glass windows and a choir loft with pipe organ. I sang in the schola (short for schola cantorum) for high Mass and took turns with another novice, also a music major, playing the organ for all Masses. It wasn't uncommon for me to get my feet tangled in the organ foot pedals and make a mess of a postlude. On balance, I enjoyed being encouraged in my musical abilities.

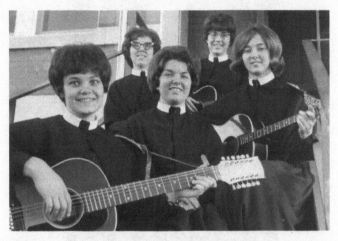

All the new postulants were pictured in the community magazine in small groups. I am in the foreground in this group with the twelve-string guitar. Next to me is Susan, a friend from high school, followed in the front row by Chris, also on guitar. Back row, left to right, Margo and Linda, also a friend from high school. (Circa late 1965)

In the convent, the bell rang when it was time for breakfast (after toilet-scrubbing duty), when it was time for lunch, and when it was time for dinner. Our main meal was at noon, which is also a healthy way to eat.

Communal meals are the times when all monks of an institution are together. Diet and eating habits differ somewhat by monastic order, and more widely by schedule. The Benedictine rule is illustrative.

The *Rule of St. Benedict* orders two meals. Dinner (lunch) is provided year-round; supper is also served from late spring to early fall, except for Wednesdays and Fridays. The diet originally consisted of simple fare: two dishes, with fruit as a third course if available; the meat of mammals was forbidden to all but the sick. Moderation in all aspects of diet is the spirit of St. Benedict's law.

Our meals were not as spartan as those of the Benedictines. We had meat, a starch, vegetables, and dessert at most meals, all very balanced and I thought pretty good. I remember a great deal of variety in the food served.

Meals were eaten in the refectory.

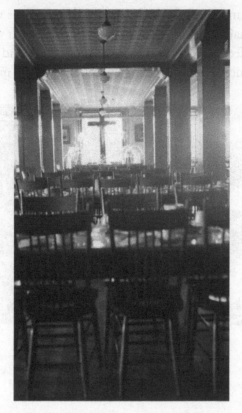

Refectory (dining room) shot back to front of room with dais, ferns, and crucifix in front

The refectory was a large basement room with small windows above the ground line and large weight-bearing square pillars strategically placed throughout the room. I remember some sort of potted ferns in the refectory, which added some warmth to an otherwise stern-looking room. The room was very brown. The wooden floors creaked (making it even more difficult to sneak around in the refectory at night). They also buckled in the summer Iowa humidity, making them hard to buff.

At the front of the room was a speaker's dais set with a small table and a chair. In front of the dais were rows and rows of tables, each one set for ten, to accommodate the approximately two hundred postulants and novices. There was a designated time to start and stop each meal, as signaled by a bell. Everything was signaled by bells.

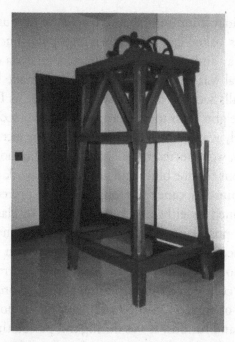

The Motherhouse Bell was originally purchased in 1856 and brought to the Motherhouse from the original location of the order at St. Joseph's Prairie, just outside of Dubuque, Iowa. The bell was used continuously while I was living at the convent in the 1960s. The bell tolled for rising and was rung 10 minutes before Mass and evening Vespers. The bell called us to meals and tolled on festive days when talking at meals was allowed. A single long gong of one of the chimes indicated a death.

Novices with kitchen duty served the platters of food. When everyone was seated and grace had been said, a professed sister would ascend the dais, open a book on the table, and begin spiritual reading aloud. I don't remember what kinds of things were read during the meal. I do remember that it was a time to eat slowly, savoring each bite, as there weren't too many bites to savor. Our concentration was also on the spiritual reading. The food was not the focus. I do remember that the readings were more or less inspiring and of interest.

Breakfast was eaten in silence. On each platter appeared five portions of whatever was being served: five paper cups of baked eggs, five slices of Spam, or five hard-boiled eggs. The opportunity for seconds occurred only when someone didn't want her portion, as I recall. In earlier, less enlightened times, seconds were available. However, no one could leave the table until all the food was finished. I think that must have made for some pretty heavy novices.

I knew on Friday mornings that I would be in business for seconds, because Friday was baked-egg day, rather unpopular fare. I liked eggs prepared any which way and was quite willing to eat an extra one if offered. Also served at every meal was a plate stacked with homemade bread. We had our own bakery, after all. Seconds of bread were available. As I was self-conscious about being overweight, I was too embarrassed to take a second piece of bread, though I desperately wanted one. No opportunity for secret eating here.

After breakfast, we reported to "All Saints" (all the rooms and dorms had saints' names) to put on our blues and get ready to work. Blues consisted of soft, light blue denim-like capes and long aprons to protect our habits.

A bell summoned us either back to duties or to classes depending on whether we were postulants (classes), canonical-year novices (duties and instruction), or second-year novices (instruction and classes at Clarke College). Instructions were given in the large novitiate room by the novice mistress. This was considered our formation period in preparation for vows. My time was one of turmoil in the Catholic Church post–Vatican II. The changes came fast and furious. It was during this period that many sisters left religious life. Older professed sisters were often bewildered by the changes.

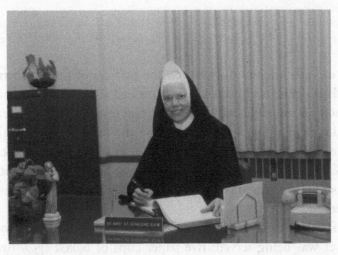

Novice Mistress, Sister Mary Geraldine, 1960s. Sister was instrumental in guiding the novices "to discover what's important in life" each morning at instructions.

Our instruction was very cutting-edge. I remember being asked questions for discussion. We were encouraged, as I remember it, to share our opinions. There was no room for old minutia. We also took classes in theology taught by a recognized theologian, Sister Joan, who later became president of the order. Discussions about theology and books by the likes of Pierre Teilhard de Chardin pushed our thinking to new levels. We explored Old and New Testament alike. We were trained, just as I had been trained in high school by this order of nuns, to appreciate our Jewish heritage. I especially enjoyed my class in comparative religions, learning about many Eastern religions as well as those of the West. We studied the history of Protestantism: Calvin and Luther. My favorite class was the one on Protestant hymn tunes, many of which have been adopted by the Catholics as the years have passed.

The bell signaled the time for before-noon meal duties. During my canonical year, that meant "Priests' Kitchen" for me. I also had a variety of other much less memorable duties during my two years in the novitiate, including buffing floors and high dusting. Many novices had kitchen duties: preparing meals, serving meals, cleaning up the kitchen. The only kitchen duty I had was Priests' Kitchen. (More about that in the next chapter.)

There would be a bell that signaled the end of the noon meal, and we would go back to work or study. When the supper bell rang, we again appeared in the refectory at our assigned tables, which we rotated periodically. Supper was the lightest meal of the day.

After supper, we indulged in a period of recreation, which might be a game of softball outside, weather permitting, or bowling down at the barn. I didn't know how to bowl, and I remember sitting at the upright piano on the lower floor of the barn below the bowling alley, playing sing-along-type tunes and show tunes on the piano. A novice or two would also hang behind and sing around the piano with me. Sometimes we sat around the novitiate singing; I and others would play the guitar. This was the height of the hootenanny days, and I knew all the Peter, Paul and Mary tunes, Dylan, and a bit of The Weavers, which harked back to an earlier time. As was apropos, one of my favorite songs to sing and play was "The Times They Are A-Changin' " by Bob Dylan.

Some evenings included vespers in the chapel, perhaps once a week. We also had choir practice on a weekly basis, as well as, for me, schola practice and organ and piano practice. I loved singing in the schola up in the choir loft, looking down on hundreds of sisters praying and singing. Evening ceremonies such as midnight Mass at Christmas were breathtaking from above: the glow from hundreds of candles carried by each sister, the processions. Evenings included study time, as I recall. We also spent time mending our socks while a professed sister would read to us from the front of the postulate or novitiate. On Sundays, we wrote letters home to our families.

Lights-out time was 9:30 p.m. The upstairs was filled with several large dorm rooms on both the second and third floors. The evening bedtime ritual included showering, of course, but also a trip to the lavatory, basin in hand, to get water for the morning ablutions. This procedure was done in silence. It was easy to fall asleep. We were physically and mentally exhausted. That 5:30 a.m. bell the next morning came all too soon.

PRIESTS' KITCHEN

My duty during our canonical year in the novitiate was Priests' Kitchen. In our order, a person was a novice for two years. The first year was the canonical year, devoted to prayer, religious instruction, and house duties. In a large convent housing several hundred sisters at any given time, a lot of help is needed to run it. In my group, there were 55 of us ready for housework upon receiving the white veil that proclaimed us novices.

I'm sure both the postulant mistress, Sister Anne Marie, whose charge we were about to leave, and the novice mistress, Sister Mary Geraldine, whose charges we were about to become, gave considerable concentration to deciding which girl should receive which duties. Some had small before-breakfast duties such as cleaning a few toilets, with other duties during the day, while those with kitchen duty prepared breakfast.

I had one all-consuming duty: Priests' Kitchen. I reported to Sister Mary Teresian after Mass and before breakfast, after breakfast, before dinner, after dinner, before supper, and after supper. Sister Teresian was in charge of preparing meals for the priests who came daily to say Mass, perform other ceremonies, hear confessions, and so forth. (I would love to have been a fly on the wall in the confessional listening to a gaggle of novices make their confessions. Had I done that, I would now have more convent pranks to report, I am sure.) She also prepared meals for guests other than priests.

Every morning after 6:30 a.m. Mass, Sister Teresian prepared breakfast for the priest who said Mass. My job was to help Sister Teresian in any way she asked. She prepared the eggs and so on for the priests. I prepared side dishes like fruit bowls and got things ready to set the table. She had to set the table herself, as the priests' dining rooms were on the professed sisters' side of the house and novices were not allowed to be there unless cleaning. I can't say that I didn't peek in to see the elegantly appointed dining rooms when Sister Teresian wasn't looking. She had a very stern manner and demeanor. She had a reputation among the novices as being tough, and Priests' Kitchen was a duty most girls prayed they wouldn't get.

I was one of the unlucky ones in my set who got that duty. However, after a while, I sensed that Sister Teresian was probably not really so stern or formidable—not because I was a head taller and at least 50 pounds heavier than her but because she really wasn't a very good actress. I learned later in life, during my long career as a Certified Financial Planner, the importance of reading people's faces and of hearing what isn't said, so to speak. As a professed sister, Sister Teresian was instructed not to talk to the novices except to give directions for completing a duty. I'm sure the thinking was that the novice mistress and her instructions should be the only influence upon the novices. No telling what weird ideas some of the professed sisters might convey inadvertently to impressionable novices, may have been the thought.

I had no interest in cooking or kitchens. The duty consisted of a lot of dishwashing and stain removal from linen cutwork tablecloths. The stain-removal technique learned in Priests' Kitchen is one I use to this day: Stretch the tablecloth with the spot centered over a large bowl, pour hot water from high above through the spot, and rub with a bar of light brown or golden soap, which was most likely Fels-Naptha and is what I use today. Every Monday I got to wash and iron all the cutwork tablecloths used during the week.

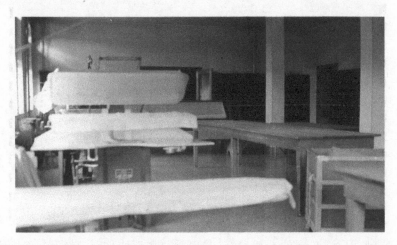

Laundry room with mangle, ironing board (where I ironed cutwork tablecloths all day every Monday), tables for folding and laying out starched head pieces, and bins (rear of picture) labeled by community number for each sister's laundry, which was all sewn with community numbers. My community number was 4744.

However, I was interested in decorating and crafts. Little did I know that this would be my joy in Priests' Kitchen. For example, a luncheon meal for guests and priests included "ribbon sandwiches," as Sister Teresian called them. This recipe often appears in cookbooks as Holiday Yule Log.

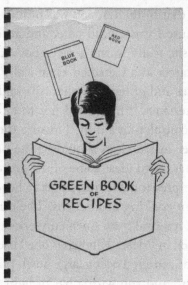

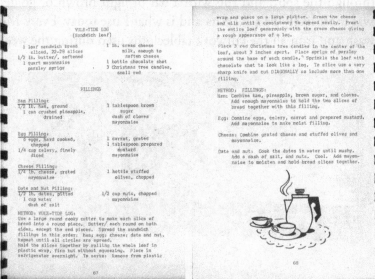

Recipe from Sister St. Clara's Green Book of Recipes for Yule-Tide Log. This is basically the recipe SM Teresian taught me to make in Priests' Kitchen. Outside of the Christmas season, this favorite was called "Ribbon Sandwiches." The top was decorated with flowers made from sliced olives, sliced bell peppers of various colors, chopped eggs and whatever else we had on hand for decorations.

Betty Crocker would have been proud of me. Crusts were cut from a loaf of bread, fillings prepared and spread, and the entire loaf was ensconced in a cream cheese coating. The best part was decorating the loaf: making flower petals out of slices of colored bell peppers, stems of green bell peppers, centers filled with shredded yellow cheese, and sliced olive borders. Part of the fun was making something decorative out of whatever ingredients were on hand.

What did Priests' Kitchen food preparation have to do with losing weight? I learned how to make a modest portion of food fill the plate using presentation. Don't we joke about this type of thing in describing servings of food presented in a fancy and expensive French restaurant? "How was dinner last night at Chez Chichi?" "Oh, we were served three peas on a white plate," and the like. Presentation is important for food satisfaction. If we are satisfied with the food in front of us, we won't feel the need to have more food. Aren't three bites of a decadent tiramisu more satisfying than a bag of meringues at 11 calories each? If we don't allow ourselves the pleasure of the tiramisu after dinner, don't we often set out upon nighttime kitchen raids eating everything in sight? (See Holy Habits #2 and #3.)

Priests' Kitchen also provided great exercise. I wasn't big on those mountain goat hikes over the hills on hot, muggy days, wearing our black cotton skirts, led by Sister Anne Marie, but hikes around the grounds with Sister Teresian in search of bittersweet in the fall and violets in the spring, with which to make floral table arrangements, were exciting. Bittersweet was wrapped around a hidden tree branch here and there. Wild violets, so small and hidden in clumps around the grounds, had us walking for probably miles without realizing we were exercising. It was all like a great Easter egg hunt for adults. Sister Teresian padded around the grounds with energy and purpose in search of wildflowers, with me in tow. I could barely keep up with her pace, amazed at her knowledge of where to find the flowers. After so much activity, how could I feel guilty about sitting with a book? I was doing something I enjoyed that involved physical activity, so why not be a guilt-free couch potato the rest of the time? (See Holy Habit #4.)

The flower arranging was done in the sacristy, as most of the flower arrangements landed on the altar in the chapel. Very conveniently, Sister Teresian was also the sacristan. The novice with sacristy duty was trained to arrange flowers, which I desperately wanted to do too. Sister Teresian invited me to the sacristy during some duty time or another and trained me in flower arranging principles, another skill I use on a regular basis to this day. I learned to make centerpieces for the elegant 18th-century-style dining rooms. I also learned to set up contemporary flower arrangements: using anchor flowers to set the form of the arrangement, and then filling in with other flowers. I could tell that Sister Teresian was pleased that she had a novice with talent for the duty.

Not long after being assigned to the duty, I embarked upon a campaign to get Sister Teresian to smile and laugh even if she couldn't really talk to me about anything more than where to put a flower and how to dry a dish. I would say things with a twinkle in my eye, like, "Why don't we sneak out, get a bus downtown, and visit a local florist to get ideas?" and "Are you going to report me to Sister Geraldine [the novice mistress] for talking to you?" I could see Sister Teresian stifling a laugh. (She never reported me, I'm sure.)

I corresponded with Sister Teresian and visited with her periodically through the ensuing years until her death on May 15, 1997. A highlight for me was taking her to lunch at Tavern on the Green, with its floral beauty in bucolic Central Park, when she came to visit me in New York City in the 1980s. This was a relationship formed with no words, only action and expression, but followed up on for years with words through correspondence.

Thinking about her reminds me of my Priests' Kitchen adventures, about how losing weight was accomplished while completing other tasks and while learning lifetime habits about food and presentation and flower arranging. I wasn't thinking about losing weight. I wasn't thinking about exercising. I do recall feeling sorry for myself upon occasion when I was still in the kitchen washing dishes after having had a lot of guests for dinner. I watched the other girls out at recreation, running around, playing games. I could see the movement of legs and feet and long black skirts through the small, high windows in the basement kitchen. I was missing recreation because I was still washing dishes. There were no dishwashers. But on balance, I had made lemonade out of what was considered a lemon of a duty called Priests' Kitchen.

MARIAN HALL AND THE SINGING NUN

It's no secret that nuns, brothers, and priests live long lives. Why is that? And while there is the occasional roly-poly nun and Santa Claus–bellied priest, for the most part those in religious life appear to be within normal weight. I can't speak for the men, but I can comment on what I observed in the convent.

As postulants, not long after we entered, we were assigned to one sister at Marian Hall, which was the community nursing home on the grounds next to the motherhouse, to visit on a regular basis. I really didn't think of Marian Hall as a nursing home. At age 18 I had no experience with nursing homes or the people in them. I had no negative preconceived notions about who and what I might find at Marian Hall. In visiting Marian Hall, I found older to elderly sisters, each in her room in various stages of alertness and health, very welcoming to me. Some were sick, and I think some were just retired and frail. Each room contained the mark and feeling of the sister in it: a colorful blanket, pictures, and knickknacks. And mostly what I remember is being greeted by a smile as I walked into each room.

I took it upon myself to go from room to room with my guitar, singing mostly folk songs. This was 1965 and the height of the hootenanny era, which I bought into big-time. It was also the time of "The Singing Nun," Soeur Sourire, a Belgian sister who topped the charts in 1963 with "Dominique." I fancied myself at once The Singing Nun and queen of the sing-along. When they were up to it, I would encourage the sisters to sing along with me. I had the Peter, Paul and Mary songbooks, the Judy Collins songbooks, the *100 Folk Songs* book containing things like "Black Is the Color of My True Love's Hair" and The Weavers classics. I had no idea that Peter, Paul and Mary, for example, had a political agenda. I just liked the songs and so did the sisters. Freedom songs, such as "Donna Donna," I copied from groups I'd heard in high school, only mimicking a message I didn't really understand. I never left a room without singing "Danny Boy," which was always the favorite. Again, I had no sense of ethnicity. I had a mother who told me, when I asked what nationality I was so I could fill it in on my high school application form, that I was "a little of everything." Little then did I realize that "Danny Boy" was an Irish song and that most of the nuns in the order were of Irish heritage. After all, the names of the girls in my own set ran like Mary Jane O'Brien, Mary Ann Fitzgerald, and Mary Sue Boyle. With the same kind of double first name, Mary Lou, and a Scottish last name, Reid, I wasn't far out of the mainstream in the order, itself founded by Irish women.

I know I spent some of my recreation time singing to the elderly at Marian Hall, but then, I didn't like sports much and was relieved not to be playing ball or some other outdoor game with the rest of the novices/postulants. I think back now and wonder if anyone missed me or wondered where I had gone. I didn't ask anyone's permission. The assignment to visit one sister at Marian Hall just expanded for me into a mission of visiting with anyone who welcomed me into her room.

The sister I was assigned to visit was very frail, very yellow, and lay in a bed with rails around it, as I recall. I had never seen anyone look like that, and learned that Sister was dying of liver cancer. I don't know that she really knew I was there. I sang to her, of course. Maybe that's why I branched out and visited other sisters; I enjoyed getting a response.

This was a new world to me. I saw food being served, basic balanced meals of modest volume. I learned much more about "food for the elderly" years later when I admitted my own mother to an assisted-living facility and ultimately to a nursing home.

At Marian Hall, there was Mass for those who could attend and other spiritual activities. I wonder if the priests visiting at Marian Hall also ate in my Priests' Kitchen at the motherhouse?

I never saw the priests or other dining room guests over whom we fussed preparing those ribbon sandwiches and fried eggs. I came to this setting with no bias or preconceived notions. Marian Hall was never referred to as a nursing home. My other regular contact with Marian Hall was again when the bell tolled throughout the grounds noting that there had been a death. I, of course, was sorry on general principle that someone had died, usually someone I didn't know personally. I was too timid to ask questions, even a name, so many of the sisters I sang to remained nameless. But the flip side of the death-toll bell for me was the realization that soon there would be a funeral Mass at Marian Hall.

As I mentioned previously, I was in the schola, which meant getting out of some duty or another to go sing for the funeral Mass. I loved singing much more than I loved housekeeping duties. From the choir loft at Marian Hall, I enjoyed watching the proceedings below. I was eternally grateful that I did not have to play the organ for the Mass, as I often did at Mount Carmel. Sister Mary Marilyn, my organ teacher at Mount Carmel, was very stern and formidable. She did not respond very well to my offhand quips. Playing the large pipe organ with its foot pedals, booming from the choir loft of the motherhouse chapel throughout the entire chapel, scared me to death. My favorite piece to play was "Sing to Yahweh a New Song" in four flats, minor key, reaching back to Old Testament sentiments. One morning I made a complete mess of a joyous postlude at the end of Mass. I kept going as if I were Johann Sebastian Bach himself. Maybe as the nuns exited the chapel, they thought I was playing some contemporary 12-tone row piece filled with dissonance. Maybe I should have stuck to singing with my guitar.

FIRED FROM THE SACRISTY AND PROMOTED TO DAY AND NIGHT KITCHEN DUTY

One novice in my set, Teri, was assigned to sacristy duty at the generalate. The generalate was the building that housed the offices and living quarters of the officers of the community. In my day, we had three sacristies: the motherhouse, Marian Hall, which was the infirmary, and the generalate. At that time, an era of no shortage of priests, we had a different priest to say Mass in each chapel simultaneously and many sisters in residence to attend each Mass. Today, while two chapels are still in use, the motherhouse and Marian Hall, Mass is alternated monthly between the chapels, as the sisters are down to one priest for all.

The generalate sacristan, Sister Mary Jane, seemed a little weird to novice Teri, mainly because she never said anything. But of course, the professed sisters 50 years ago did not talk to the young novices except in the few words it took to communicate the instructions needed to complete the duty. And then again, what seemed "weird" to a typical 19-year-old girl may not really have been weird. Despite good intentions, Teri broke a steam iron and dropped a vigil lamp in one day, which caused her to be fired from sacristy duty. Teri was reassigned to the kitchen. Teri already spent her night duty in the kitchen, and now she would be there in the daytime too. Teri's fate was now day and night kitchen duty.

The sister in charge of the kitchen, Grace Ann, was a registered dietitian, but most importantly, she was a lot of fun. Teri was probably grateful to have been fired from sacristy duty. Things went smoothly for Teri in the kitchen—until Grace Ann was out one day and left the day's menus for the novices to prepare. The dessert scheduled on the menu was butterscotch pudding. Teri always thought that the butterscotch pudding tasted like sawdust, so she and the other novices decided to "improve" it. First, they added four gallons of whipped cream. Understand that these girls were preparing dessert for about three hundred nuns. That addition didn't seem to do much, so they tossed in a commercial-sized bag of chocolate chips, which Teri thought improved matters a bit. I guess I ate the pudding served, but then, I ate anything. Grace Ann returned home none the wiser.

Sister Teri is now serving her second term as president of the congregation. I wonder if the electorate knew about the sister's being fired from sacristy duty and the butterscotch pudding creation.

SISTER MARY ALMA AND THE CELERY CAPER

One of Sister Mary Alma's duties as a novice was to report to the vegetable room to peel carrots, cut up potatoes, wash celery, and perform other similar tasks. I don't remember the vegetable room, but Mary Alma was a novice some 15 years ahead of me. In fact, I first met Sister Mary Alma as Sister Mary Robert Emmett, when I was in high school. Sister was my homeroom, religion, English, and journalism teacher in junior year. What I most remember about my days in journalism, besides the fascination with writing for the school paper, were the hours after school spent in the press room learning to play the ukulele. Sister Mary Robert Emmett (SMRE) was my informal ukulele teacher. The small group of us all played soprano ukes, the ones that look like toys. I soon invested in a baritone ukulele, strung like the top four strings of a guitar, a larger instrument with a richer sound. By the time I entered the convent, I was playing a Gibson 12-string guitar. Following that action plan, I guess you could say SMRE taught me to play the guitar. On the side, I learned a bit about journalism too.

Back to the vegetable room. One day a fellow novice—and I'm sure about this from knowing SMRE, a fellow conspirator in occasional pranks—and SMRE headed to the vegetable room. A third novice and friend of these two girls, Sister Donna, wasn't feeling well. SMRE and her cohort wanted to cheer up Sister Donna. It seems that Sister Donna just loved celery. Who loves celery? Only thin people.

I ask SMRE, "Is Sister Donna a thin person?"

"Yes, as I recall," says SMRE.

While SMRE and the fellow novice are in the process of selecting the perfect bunch of celery to take to Sister Donna, in walks Sister Mary Attracta, a rather elderly retired sister born in Ireland. Her duties in retirement included a little bit of dusting around the refectory (as we called the dining room then), kitchen, and vegetable room. At the sight of Sister Mary Attracta, SMRE quickly hides the celery under the top cape portion of her habit. Unless SMRE had suddenly grown lumpy, celery-shaped breasts, she was clearly hiding something. Did Sister Mary Attracta say anything to the young novices who were clearly where they didn't belong at that time of day? Perhaps the novices should have been in prayer and meditation or even at recreation, but not in the vegetable room. Were the girls scolded by Sister Mary Attracta?

Nothing was said, but of course SMRE's fears didn't end there. 65 years ago, the professed sisters did not engage in conversation with novices. The job of instructing young novices was that of the novice mistress. The big question: Would Sister Mary Attracta report SMRE to the novice mistress? SMRE was sure she was going to be sent home the next day for the celery caper. (By the way, the bunch of celery *did* cheer up Sister Donna. Mission accomplished.) Days passed and SMRE heard nothing. Had Sister Mary Attracta reported the incident to Sister Leo, novice mistress? Was it possible Sister Leo wouldn't call SMRE into her office for a scolding at best and dismissal from the convent at worst? Did Sister Mary Attracta keep the whole thing to herself?

The answer to those questions is unknown, but we do know this: As it happens, an Irish rebel who fought against the British at the turn of the 19th century was named Robert Emmet[1].

While it might be fitting for SMRE to be named after a rebel, her religious name, Robert Emmett (extra "t" added on the end for distinction from the rebel), was the given name of one of Mary Alma's brothers. Mary Alma came from a good Irish family, and with a name like Robert Emmett, would Mary Alma be favored by Sister Mary Attracta, a fellow Irishwoman, or would she be betrayed? Mary Alma believes that Sister Mary Attracta probably kept the whole incident to herself.

Mary Alma lives happily ever after to this day as a sister, and ever a rebel.

---

[1]   Robert Emmet (March 4, 1778–September 20, 1803) was an Irish nationalist and Republican, orator, and rebel leader. (Wikipedia) After leading an abortive rebellion against British rule in 1803 he was captured, then tried and executed for high treason against the British king. He came from a wealthy Anglo-Irish Protestant family who sympathized with Irish Catholics and their lack of fair representation in Parliament. The Emmet family also sympathized with the rebel colonists in the American Revolution. While Emmet's efforts to rebel against British rule failed, his actions and speech after his conviction inspired his compatriots.

ELLEN AND THE TREAT CUPBOARD: LETTERS HOME TELL THE TRUTH ABOUT CONVENT FOOD

Ellen was in my set, which means she entered the convent with me on July 31, 1965. Ellen sparks a ray of sunshine wherever she goes, because she wears a smile that just won't quit. This was so in 1965, and the same is true today. Ellen is no longer a nun.

When I tell people that I lost 50 pounds in the convent, one of the first things I'm asked is, "Was the food that bad?" For me the food was varied and tasty, but then, my mother was a terrible cook. Ellen also enjoyed the convent food.

Ellen's mother kept all 72 letters Ellen wrote home in those early postulant and novitiate years, so here is actual testimony, excerpts from Ellen's letters written over 50 years ago, mentioning the food quite often with lots of "yum, yum." Ellen is and was a foodie. These excerpts span only her first two months in the convent.

August 6, 1965: "It seems like every time we turn around we're eating. I'm not complaining (you can be sure). The food is great and plentiful.... The past two nights we've had picnic suppers outside because the weather has been so nice....There is a popcorn machine in the barn..."

August 15, 1965: "Yesterday we were two weeks old as postulants...Can you believe it? The novices baked a delicious cake for us....Phoebe, Mary, and I received a big package from Peg and Nancy. They sent us a big box of Fanny Farmer chocolates. Yum!"

August 16, 1965: "We've been having picnic suppers every night because of the beautiful evenings we've been having. Last night we brought our supper way out to the hills and afterward had a hootenanny. It was such a beautiful night...."

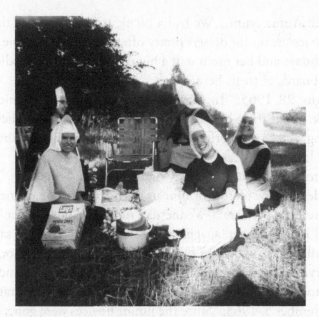

Out for a picnic on the grounds on a warm summer day, circa 1966. Left to right: Professed Sister Mary Teresian, in charge of Priest's kitchen where I worked as well as the sacristy; Marybeth wearing "blues" to save the serge habit; a prominent box of Lay's Potato Chips, a diet favorite; Mira, daring in her sartorial style without cape, rolled up sleeves and blues apron; Mary Lou, author, in full blues apron; and Kristine, also in blues apron. Blues were made of a light cotton material in a light denim blue color, worn for work and play. I still see friends Mira and Kristine on a regular basis. Mira is still a BVM and recently completed two terms as first Vice-President of the order.

A little ways beyond the convent is the apple orchard. There are tons of apples all over the place, and so-o-o good to eat."

- August 18, 1965: "We always have our big meal at noon. You wouldn't believe how good the food is…just like home cooking. Sister Grace Ann is in charge of the cooking."
- August 20, 1965: "This place sure does know how to get rid of left-overs…gag….What we don't eat for breakfast and lunch, we find on the table for supper, with a few minor physical changes of course. We can often predict what the next meal will be….It's great fun, choke, choke!….We have an apple orchard with wonderful apples and a ton of big red tomatoes so consequently we find a zillion different forms of both on our plates each day—examples: apple pie, apple sauce, apple streusel crunch, apple cake, and so on; stuffed tomatoes, stewed tomatoes, fresh tomatoes, tomatoes in salads and

sauce. Yum...yum...We had a picnic tonight out past the barn. We have ice cream for dessert pretty often!....Today was one of the girls' birthdays and her mom sent a big cake and tons of goodies. We have cupboards of treats here."

- August 28, 1965: "Tuesday night, the novices had a picnic at Murphy Park, about three blocks away from Mount Carmel. They invited us along. It was wonderful—lots of food!! It was the first time any of us had left Mount Carmel."

- September 1, 1965: "Sunday night we went to the barn. The novices made big bins of popcorn for us in the popcorn machine...yum!!"

- September 4, 1965: "Wednesday night the novices cooked a beautiful Italian supper: spaghetti, meatballs, Italian bread, salad, cheese, candlelight, soda water, butterscotch brownies with chocolate chips; everything except wine. It was delicious! The novices and postulants sat together for this meal too. Ordinarily we sit at separate tables."

- September 5, 1965: "Since the junior novices were gone, some of the postulants made a picnic supper—it was the best picnic we had!.... My package arrived this morning—thanks for everything. The kids are eating the toffee now. It's the best toffee I've ever tasted—yum. We have a huge cupboard filled with the candy people send. Some of it is put out each afternoon."

- September 12, 1965: "Labor Day was really excellent. The novices fixed the novitiate up like an espresso coffee house. They had modern art, colored spotlights, small tables with wine bottles, candles and lots of room on the floor to sit and eat our pizzas and Coke. The name of the house was 'the Fickle Pickle,' complete with entertainment. We were literally rolling on the floor....Yesterday I was among some of the postulants who made apple jelly. It was fun....Can you see us running around the kitchen not knowing where anything is, singing, talking, laughing? Poor Sister Mary. Grace Ann putting up with us and helping with her wonderful humor. The result was delicious (despite how sick of apples we are). Our family couldn't go through all the jelly we made in a year. We make things in large quantities here. The first thing I did wrong was open one of the cupboards and the door fell off!!"

- October 2, 1965—"For our supper tonight we went on about a five-mile hike to Julian Dubuque's grave. The view of the Mississippi is breathtaking! It was the best weather we have had since we've been here. Perfect fall weather."

- Little did Ellen know when she delighted in the treat cupboard during those first days in the convent that her next duty would be director of the treat cupboard.
- September 25, 1965: "Yesterday our duties were changed and my new one is cleaning a small room named 'G.' It contains art supplies, treats, and other odds and ends. I also have the popular task of passing out treats every afternoon....Everyone thinks I'll get much fatter...hope not!"

Ellen's weight fate was sealed...a nibble here, a nibble there while arranging the chocolates....We all know that story! While preparing nightly dinner we taste the gravy, swallow a spoonful of stuffing to see if it needs more salt, lick the cake frosting off the beaters...and 15 more pounds later we don't know what happened. I'm afraid "everyone" was right: Ellen put on 15 pounds as a postulant and soon had to let out her black skirt at the waist.

Did the postulant mistress know that by putting Ellen in charge of the treat cupboard, she was putting the fox in charge of the henhouse? The treat cupboard was a large built-in Victorian cabinet, and it was the storehouse for the goodies in "G." (The rooms along the postulant corridor had letter names, and in fact that corridor, now remodeled into rooms for retired sisters, is called "Letter Wing.") The treat cupboard had tall, heavy, sliding wooden doors and contained a large stash of the best and most expensive boxes of chocolates: See's, Fanny Farmer, Fanny May, Godiva, all from doting parents in celebration of a daughter's birthday and holidays. There was no shortage of birthdays and no shortage of treats. With each box devoured, new inventory arrived to take its place. Nothing was kept individually, but rather turned in to the superior to be shared by all, hence the existence of the treat cupboard.

My parents never sent candy, and I don't think it was because I was overweight. My parents, ever the practical sort, sent things like those fleece pajamas with feet for warm sleeping in the drafty old Motherhouse.

Happily for the other girls, most parents did not send pajamas. The highlight of the day for many was the 1 p.m. treat buffet after class. Ellen was never at a loss for helpers because, of course, helpers got first dibs on the best candy choices.

Ellen shared the following about how she felt as "captain" of the treat cupboard in 1965: "I often felt I was out in the world and worked in the storeroom of a downtown candy shop, eyeing up the strong stacks of neat white boxes waiting to be sampled. As an added benefit to the daily work of sweeping and dusting the ancient room I would ease my homesickness with a delectable morsel or two, to savor while I cleaned."

There's a happy ending to this 15-pound weight-gain story. Ellen soon became a junior novice and therefore was no longer in charge of the treat cupboard. Lots of house duties came with being a junior novice, which meant lots of "accidental" exercise. After a year in the novitiate, which included not only house duties but also well-balanced meals, fewer snacks, and lots of *Sound of Music*–style hikes, songs, and climbing the hills on the grounds, Ellen lost 25 pounds. She hadn't been this thin in a long time, she shared. 52 years later, Ellen confesses still to an eternal weakness for chocolate, though as I look at Ellen now, I don't see much of it settled around her middle! Looks like Ellen has carried those slimming novitiate habits with her through the years, while of course, always eating dessert.

PART II

GETTING INTO THE HABITS

The Importance of Creating Habits

Restaurant critic and cookbook author Nigella Lawson has said, "Food is about memories. It's rich and messy and anarchic—much like life." We are probably more familiar with the term "anarchy" as it relates to governments and battles. But our relationship with food is truly "without order" and often chaotic as well. We cannot divorce food and remain single as we might with a spouse or friends. We must eat to survive. How do we bring order to the sometimes chaotic food choices we make? Or is it just too difficult? Wouldn't it be nice if we could bring order to our food choices and then let them remain on autopilot while we concentrated on the other activities of life? We *can* do just that. In life, it often seems so easy to set ourselves up for failure. Why shouldn't it be just as easy to set ourselves up for success?

Setting good eating habits on autopilot is really another way of saying: Don't think about food, just live your life. The autopilot way of dealing with food may take some time in the beginning. It also takes time in the beginning to practice a new relationship with food so that it becomes a habit. It's in the first two steps that most people fail: 1) creating a new habit and 2) practicing that habit. Did I enjoy practicing the piano between lessons as a child? Did Mickey Mantle[2] get out in the field and practice baseball every day or just dream of becoming a professional ballplayer like Babe Ruth? So, we must ask ourselves, how much do we really want to succeed in creating new eating habits?

---

[2]   Mickey Mantle was a New York Yankees Hall of Fame baseball player from 1951 to 1968; he ranks 18th of all time in home runs, with 536.

When we were age five, when presented with a new two-wheeler bike, how motivated were we to graduate from a tricycle to a grown-up two-wheeler? The bike often came with training wheels and perhaps with the help of a parent. I remember clearly the gray-blue 20-inch Schwinn bike with white sidewall tires and streamers on the handles that appeared in the yard for my fifth birthday. I couldn't wait to get out and try riding the bike. Of course, I was frightened too. Seeing the training wheels was comforting. My fear was overcome by my desire to ride a two-wheeled bike. I remember so clearly that moment, without training wheels, with my father running alongside me, holding the bike. Then he let go—and I kept riding! That sentence tells the story of my life.

I've always been a fearful introvert. I drove my mother nuts saying, "What if...?" to everything, looking at all possible negative options. But I was also driven by the desire to succeed at things. I was always rewarded for success and encouraged to try things, but I was never scolded for failure. I was rewarded for having *tried* no matter the outcome. Failure in our house was seen simply as the next step on the path to success. As a timid, introverted, and fearful child, I was always coaxed and encouraged and rewarded for effort. I was not encouraged to get straight As in school but to do my best—because I put so much pressure on myself to get straight As and was so deflated to get a B in something that I didn't want to bring home the report card. My parents treated a report card containing a B the same as one with all As: "Good job."

I entered the convent, as noted, after high school. I brought with me my idealism and enthusiasm. I also brought with me not a whole lot of self-confidence or self-worth, not unusual for someone 17 years old. In the convent, I found other girls with similar combinations of confidence, fear, and uncertainty, who were short, tall, thin, heavy, attractive, and not so attractive. Our "formation" included plenty of things to inspire a positive self-worth and positive self-talk, though in those days the conversation didn't include such words and terms. We were not mired in the minutia that may have colored convent training in earlier days: "After you clean the floors, be sure to get the chairs put back in the exact spot where they belong again, as marked by the tape." No one seemed to notice or care that I was overweight. I began to grow inside instead of outside.

This is where I first learned the positive self-talk that has stayed with me throughout my life. Maybe my parents saved a lot of money on psychiatrists by allowing me to enter the convent. I have heard others say that they had to go see a psychiatrist after their years in the convent. But then, this is *my* story.

Similarly, when it comes to changing an eating habit, there must be focus and practice applied in the beginning. Failure must be seen as one more step taken on the road to success. And reward yourself for a B as much as for an A. We are not looking for perfection, as my husband reminds me often, just improvement.

How does this relate to eating in the convent, you might ask? The job there was easier because food, like everything else, was out of our control. I had my eating habits changed *for* me. And those habits were reinforced for two and a half years, after which time the new way of eating was truly a habit for me. However, I've had to maintain the eating habits learned in the convent for the past 45 years without the structure of the convent. How did I do that?

Changing an eating habit requires some soul-searching. I cannot recommend that everyone enter a convent or the monastic priesthood to be controlled "from above" by some version of religious food rules. The question remains: How can we create order out of food anarchy and have enough self-control to create new habits for ourselves and live by them? This is a tall order.

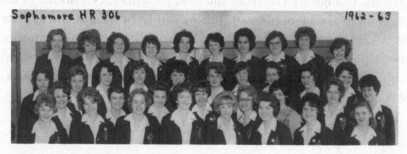

My sophomore homeroom class at Our Lady of Peace High School. I'm on the right end of the third row smiling with a chubby face. (1962-63)

What eating habits were reinforced in your childhood? Were you required to clean your plate because there were starving children in China who were not as lucky as you to be given three squares a day? Maybe you would have loved to tell your mother to send those ugly lima beans over to the starving children in Asia. That was probably not an option if you didn't want to be sent to your room with no supper. Were you served pasta for lunch and dinner? In our house the real favorite was Campbell's Spaghetti-Os. We were also the first on our block to eat Swanson's fried chicken TV dinners. (This was the 1950s.) One of my jobs upon arriving home from high school at about 6 p.m. (I lived a long way from my school) was to choose a canned vegetable for dinner, open the can, pour the peas into the pot, and heat them up. Yum, yum—I got to select a side dish of salty pale peas for dinner! The worst for me was smelling the salmon croquets made of canned salmon baking in the oven, just waiting to be topped with gummy pea sauce. My mother was a terrible cook, though meals were balanced and included a serving each of meat, starch, salad, and vegetable.

We all have our stories. I pigged out on potato chips and dip after dinner because I ate only a small portion of the meat, baked to a frazzle and accompanied by canned vegetables at dinner. That's an example of figuring out one of the "whys" of becoming overweight. Making up for an unsatisfying dinner by eating a pound of potato chips and dip afterwards wasn't a good solution to the problem. I now see the problem, and that's 90 percent of the battle. Back then, I was a child under the control of my parents. Am I going to blame my mother for bad cooking and my father (who was overweight) for bad genes, saying, "Oh, well, it's somebody else's fault that I'm overweight"?

At some point, we must take control of our own lives. We can't blame our parents, though we can recall the food patterns they instilled in us as a reason. We can't bemoan the past, but we can learn from it and address the future. We can't say, "I've lived this way for so long; I can't change now." It's always possible to change and do whatever it is in life we really want to do. Colonel Sanders first franchised Kentucky Fried Chicken at age 62, for heaven's sake!

Is Routine Enslaving or Is It Freeing?

N
ow that I'm motivated to create good food habits, what do I do?
Many of us follow a busy work routine, come home and put on the homemaker apron, fall into bed exhausted, and start all over again the next day. We feel like a rat in a maze. Sound familiar? Our lives are routine and stultifying. Is this routine something foisted upon us by others? Have we lost ourselves in the process? If this is the case, routine is indeed enslaving.

Let's look at another type of routine. This routine may well contain some or all of the same elements, but this one is created by *me*. If not totally created by me, it's at least one I have proactively chosen. It's one to which I have said yes. I think of the TV show *Say Yes to the Dress* as a simple tangible example of something we can apply to intangible concepts such as life choices. In the show *Say Yes to the Dress*, we see half an hour in the life of a bride-to-be as she goes through the process of choosing a wedding gown. By the end of the program, the bride says yes to the dress of her choice. The bride always comes to the salon with an entourage: friends, mother, grandmother, and/or mother of the groom. She is looking for approval, for help sharing the decision-making process. In some cases, she even leaves the decision to one or all of her advisors. In other cases, she makes her own decision, overriding the no's of her advisors. The decision always sticks when it comes from the bride, with or without the approval of others. A decision from the heart makes for a happy bride. A routine created in the heart of the person following it is a freeing routine. We must consciously say yes to the routine.

A self-chosen routine gives you the freedom to focus on other things. At Mount Carmel, we followed a routine. Granted, the details of the routine were not chosen by the individual sisters. But the decision to follow the routine of a chosen religious order was indeed very personal and therefore freeing. The day was filled with scheduled work. But the day was also filled with scheduled personal time, scheduled prayer and meditation, and scheduled socializing. We were playing volleyball or singing show tunes around the piano, feeling no guilt that we should be finishing other projects. This was the time for play; it was part of the routine. Meals were also scheduled. The food served was scheduled. There was no guilt about eating that piece of homemade apple pie topped with cheese. The pie was part of a meal plan designed by a dietitian with our well-being in mind.

A food routine set up by the person following it is freeing. It can be done even when part of the day includes a routine set by others, such as an eight-hour-a-day job. A food routine can be followed even if travel is a large part of your days and weeks. Is the only food available on the run at the airport a burger and fries? Of course not. I keep prepackaged baggies of trail mix and nuts handy in my purse so that I'm not forced to grab a vending machine candy bar or bag of chips. I hate eating any old thing full of calories because I'm hungry and have nothing with me to eat. I don't "hold out" for long hours not eating, either, because then when I do eat, I want to eat everything in sight. Never works.

When I read about diet plans that involve too much preplanning and special foods, I lose interest. I can't do that for the long term, and I don't really believe in short-term diets. The exception to that is when I've had too many meals out with wine and can't button my skirt, I eat low-fat TV dinners for a couple of nights, cut out the wine, and go easy on the desserts. That's as close as I can come to a diet. (I had a good friend who was selling a liquid diet program using multilevel marketing, so I bought it for a while, more out of friendship than anything else. It worked short-term.)

You do not have to count calories, worry about the size of the pie slice— or even worry about eating the piece of pie. It's all part of a prearranged plan. That prearranged plan is to be followed until it becomes a habit. Just as those of us in the convent wore the same religious habit every day, keeping us from having to make wardrobe decisions, those who follow a food plan don't have to decide what to eat. It frees us to go about the important business of life.

THE REAL WORK OF LIFE

What is the real work of life? What does our life's work have to do with weight maintenance and routine?

The real work of life is not about, as Dolly Parton sang so well, "working 9 to 5." The real work of life is about completing the urgent things in our day in time to get to the important ones, which are what really matter to each of us. Do you find your day so filled with urgent phone calls—"Can you come over and sit with my son Johnny while I take daughter Susie to the emergency room because she fell on some shards of glass?" and the like—that you can't find time to do what's important to you? Sometimes it takes time, energy, and thought to even decipher what's important to each of us.

The ordered convent life provided the time and focus to discover "the important." There were designated times for meditation, for prayer, for recreation with others, for reading and study of all types, for writing to family, for creativity. And yes, mealtimes were ordered too.

Every morsel of food eaten was not the focus of the day; it was just a regular part of the daily order. Have you ever tried to monitor every bite you put in your mouth, feeling fully focused on losing weight, only to discover at the end of the week that you gained two pounds? "How could that be?" you ask. Weight maintenance is not a weekly job. It is part of the real work of life. It is something to work at daily and something to put on the back burner while we focus on accomplishing what is really important to us. When our days are ordered and we have taken at least a few minutes to focus on something important to us, we don't have time to focus on every morsel of food in front of us. We simply eat our meals as planned. After all, the real concern of the day is perhaps 1) to create a new marketing piece for the family business, 2) to volunteer at the kids' school or a hospital, or 3) to practice that third movement of Beethoven's "Moonlight" Sonata. How can I think about loading my plate with French fries when I have Beethoven on my plate for today?

If we don't know the real work of our life and don't take the time to identify our life's work, we have too much time to eat French fries. Life in the convent encouraged the discovery of my real life's work. My life's work in the convent included both the tangible—as in, practicing to become a fine pianist—and the intangible—as in, becoming a more centered and caring person. My talent for playing the piano was encouraged. I was sent to the Clarke College campus to study music while the other girls in my set took all their classes from teachers who came to Mount Carmel to instruct us in the basic college courses. I was encouraged to practice. But it was worth it. I don't remember wishing I had had an evening snack even once during the two and a half years I was in the novitiate. I was doing my life's work.

How many of us overeat when we are unhappy, such as working 9-to-5 at a dead-end job? Or when we are under stress—as in, the spouse, kids, and boss all seem to demand 100 percent of our time and energy? Or when we are spending our days doing only the urgent—as in, "The plants on the balcony all blew over in the windstorm today, so I must stop everything to clean up the mess"? Don't stress here; a discussion on how to handle stress is ahead.

How do you change this chaos called life? Create your own convent schedule and make sure those around you know that it is as sacred and as required as your 9-to-5 job and your family. No one will even remember the next day what was yesterday's "urgent." This is harder to do than just declaring it to be so. And of course, most of us don't live in a utopia. We need to show up at the job because we need the income. We need to do our part to create a healthy family life, and we need to put out the daily fires to avoid an obliterating explosion.

You can start doing your life's work one hour at a time. For starters, you may need an outside framework in which to "fill in the boxes" of your own life. Let's take that convent schedule and see how well it works outside of the convent.

CONVENT SCHEDULE

5:30 a.m.: Rise and dress
6 a.m.: Meditation
6:30 a.m.: Mass
7 a.m.: Morning duty and breakfast
8:30 a.m.: College studies, teaching, religious instruction, and so on
Noon: Meal
1 p.m.: After-dinner duty, more classes, study, teaching
4 p.m.: Duties, prepare supper, eat supper, spiritual reading, dish duty
6:30 p.m.: Recreation, play softball, read, sew, practice piano
9:30 p.m.: Lights out

SAMPLE PERSONAL SCHEDULE MODELED ON CONVENT SCHEDULE

6 a.m.: Rise before everyone else in the house
6:15 a.m.: Quiet meditation/thought (my time)

6:30 a.m.: Family rises, gets dressed, has breakfast; kids off to school, and so on

7:30 a.m.: Morning walk and dress for work (my time)

8:30 a.m.: Leave for work

Noon: Brown-bag it and include half-hour walk (my time)[3]

6 p.m.: Arrive home, cook and eat dinner, do dishes, kids' homework and bedtime

8:30 p.m.: Personal time with spouse, time to be a couch potato, and the like (my time)

10 p.m.: Snack and bed

Discuss "permission" to create your own schedule and follow it. At Mount Carmel, the schedule was created for us, so of course it was okay with "the powers that be." Write more about making your new schedule okay with family and friends. In the financial services business, we tell clients to think, "After me you come first." We advise clients to take care of themselves first, as in, "Spend your kids' inheritance." The same is true on a daily basis that is true on an estate-planning basis. As the cliché goes, "If Mama's not happy, nobody's happy." If you take care of yourself first, you will be a better employee, a better spouse and mother, and maybe even a thinner person!

The Seven Holy Habits will help guide you through the process of creating your own food routine, your own good eating habits, and your own positive relationship to food.

---

[3] Find time during the day, maybe at lunch, for a quick read or a walk around the block. Brown-bag it for lunch three days a week to save money, calories, and time.

Tenacity...but What Should I Eat?

How do I create a food routine and stick with it? What do I eat?
The simple answer is: Eat anything.

It's always easier to stick with a food program if the food you are eating makes sense to you. Let's talk about food as your friend first, using breakfast as an example.

Most people cannot afford to order prepared diet food from a company or pay a lot of money for "only organic," and most people do not want to eat only bananas. The Convent Diet is for everyone, even if you are on food stamps. Of course, having lots of fresh fruits and vegetables is wonderful, but if such things are unavailable or unaffordable, that's okay. The important thing is to stay the course within whatever means you have available to you. Make your own food schedule using the foods you know, like, and can afford; just eat a few bites less of them at each meal. The Seven Holy Habits will provide information, guidance, and support.

For some reason, breakfast is the meal I most remember eating in the novitiate, maybe because to this day I enjoy breakfast, or maybe because many dietitians tell us breakfast is the most important meal of the day, or maybe because it was simply easy to remember. In the convent, we had hard-boiled eggs on Monday, a slice of Spam on Tuesday, scrambled eggs on Wednesday, a slice of Spam on Thursday, and baked eggs on Friday. All entrée items were accompanied by homemade bread and some sort of fruit. It was impossible to prepare toast for two hundred women, and I really missed having hot toast for breakfast, but the bread was yummy. I grew up in a household where Wonder Bread was the norm.

On the surface, one slice of Spam, one egg, and one slice of homemade bread don't sound very low-fat. They are not. But if your usual serving of eggs is three eggs and you eat only one egg, as we did in the convent, won't you lose weight? If you wouldn't dream of eating Spam so you eat your usual breakfast meat, which is three pork sausages, are you eating more healthfully? Let's start with the calories. Two ounces of Spam have 180 calories. Two ounces of pork sausage have 190 calories. If you multiply by three, that's 570 calories for three sausages. Something like chicken sausage, at less than 100 calories, might be a better breakfast meat choice than either Spam or pork sausage based on calories. Chicken sausage may be a healthier choice than the other two as well, but if Spam is what's available and affordable to you, then so be it. You can still lose weight and be healthy; just buy the low-sodium version of Spam.

Let's talk about those eggs and use Jimmy Dean brand of low-fat breakfast sandwiches, which are made with egg whites, as an example. The regular Jimmy Dean breakfast sandwiches are made with whole eggs. For the approximately 20-calorie difference in the sandwiches, I'd rather go with the whole egg version, as it helps me feel full longer. There is more protein in a whole egg than there is in an egg white. What good is it if you're still hungry after having eaten the egg-white version and you proceed to microwave a second sandwich?

It's not necessary to go to the extreme to lose weight and be healthy. What's wrong with eating a whole egg for breakfast instead of three egg whites? The whole egg provides more protein and is less wasteful. Of course, if your doctor feels there is too much cholesterol for you in the whole egg, follow your doctor's orders. Full-fat yogurt can also be okay if it means you will actually eat yogurt. Just watch out for sugar content.

IF AT FIRST YOU DON'T SUCCEED, TRY AND TRY AGAIN

It's okay to give reasons for falling off the wagon, so to speak, for abandoning the routine, from forgetting the schedule. What we call excuses for being overweight are merely reasons for being overweight. There is some validity in all reasons, if only because they are "reasonable" to each of us. It's just that those reasons cannot become our excuses.

Do any of these sound familiar?

"I can't afford fresh vegetables or free-range chicken." We ate a lot of canned veggies and some meatless meals in the convent. I lost weight. I'm a healthy adult.

"I don't have time to shop for fresh food and cook nutritious meals." Perhaps that's because you are working and could possibly use nutritious prepared food occasionally. I often fix extra servings of healthy food when I have time to cook and freeze the extra as portions to use when I'm too busy to cook.

"I don't have time to fix a brown-bag lunch before I go to the office. I have a big family to get off to school, and so on. I just grab a candy bar and chips from the vending machines near the water cooler." One day in fresh-man year of high school, I told Sister Mary John Thomas that I hadn't had time to do my homework because I had to take two buses and walk a mile to get home from school every night, which on average took me two hours. Sister quietly said, "We always find the time to do the things we really want to do."

"I inherited 'fat genes,' so fate is against me." Genetics do play a role in whether we tend to be heavy or thin. I'm not a geneticist, so I can't speak scientifically about this topic. However, I do discuss the ectomorph, endo-morph, and mesomorph body builds in the chapter on Holy Habit #1, Visualization: You're Thin Until You're Thin. I have not read any scientific evidence showing that just because I have fat parents, I have to be fat. My brother David and I inherited "fat genes" and were both chubby kids. We are both slim adults.

"I'm traveling all the time." Airports sell shrink-wrapped chicken wraps just like they sell burgers and fries.

Whine, whine, whine [about whatever it is]. As my brother David says, "Whiners never win, and winners never whine."

A healthy, centered, and focused person, at some point, takes responsi-bility for himself or herself. Perhaps our parents screwed us up as kids and that's why we're screwy adults. At some point, we have to stop and say, "Time to take charge of my own life and move forward as the real me—not the screwed-up one my parents created." Screwy parents can be a reason but are not an excuse for being a screwy adult.

The Seven Holy Habits in this book will help you look at yourself hon-estly and hopefully enable you to make good decisions going forward.

BUT I'M HUNGRY

Feeling hungry is a problem when you are trying to lose weight and keep it off. In the convent, it didn't really matter if you felt the craving for a bedtime snack, as the refrigerators were locked. We didn't think about being hungry because there was no recourse for the problem…unless you were one of the girls bold enough to sneak downstairs and rummage around the kitchen to see if there was anything to be had. That was not me.

Unfortunately, in the real world, the refrigerator in the kitchen is not locked. Many diet books talk about using various types of distractions. Let's be real: Nothing works. If you feel hungry, you *crave* something to eat and have visions of cookies, peanut butter, and ice cream floating through your head, but no Sugar Plum Fairy. What should you do? Indulge! *How* you indulge does depend a bit upon the person. For me, even though I have dessert at dinnertime, I eat a bit of what I'm craving: a chocolate Dove square or two, a large teaspoon or two of peanut butter, or a bite or two of Babybel cheese. I would rather have exactly what I crave but in moderation than run around the kitchen eating diet potato chips, carrot sticks, or a hard-boiled egg only to feel dissatisfied. In the end, I will eat the chips, carrot sticks, and hard-boiled egg *plus* the Dove squares, peanut butter, and cheese! Why not just cut to the chase and eat the good stuff, avoiding the calories in diet chips, carrots, and hard-boiled eggs?

Many people tell me that they cannot stop at one or two of whatever it is. For example, one bag of diet chips becomes the whole box, containing six bags of chips. My advice here is to get your fix. If you need to eat the whole box of chips to feel satisfied and get over the craving, then do it. Two *good* things will happen: 1) There will be no more chips in the cupboard to eat the next night, and if you're a busy person like I am, you won't run out to the store to buy more, and 2) you will get over the craving for the time being. The key here: *Do not feel guilty.* The only way successful weight loss and *maintenance* can work is to remove the word "guilt" from your vocabulary.

We are not talking about losing ten pounds in ten days here. We are talking about a lifestyle for a lifetime. No one is perfect. Once you stuff yourself with those six bags of chips, feel satisfied and move on; you will not crave chips the next night, most likely. You will probably crave nothing the next night. Should you crave a tub of ice cream the next night, well then, a bit of discipline and self-control will be required. Eat only half the tub. The big lesson I learned about gradually eating less is that it gradually took less food to fill me up. After that night of eating all six bags of chips in the box, the next time you have such a craving, stop after eating only five bags, and so on until you are satisfied with only five bags. Eventually, most of the time, one bag will do it for you.

This will take time. The Convent Diet is not the wonder diet of the day; it is a forever lifestyle. This start-up process I describe probably cannot happen without some pain. It's worth it. All or nothing doesn't work because it creates feelings of deprivation, which eventually or quickly result in a lifetime of overeating. At this point in my life I never crave all six bags of chips in the box at one time. I usually eat one but if I want more I eat two—I, who used to eat two bags of chips from a large box of Old Dutch Potato Chips plus a 16-ounce tub of onion dip to go with the chips.

Now, after pigging out on chips, even if you give in on night two and eat a tub of ice cream, *do not give up. Do not feel guilty*...do not pass "Go" and collect two hundred dollars, as they say when playing Monopoly. We are talking about making changes that will last a lifetime, not a game of Monopoly. There is always day three, day four, week two, or week three. Start again. The icebox police do not live at your house. Remember: Your goal is not to apply for a job as a fashion model next month. Many fashion models have their own problems with food, so consider yourself to be better off than they are anyway.

Correct self-talk is crucial when it comes to nighttime refrigerator raids. Never scold yourself or feel guilty. As Scarlet O'Hara said, "I'll think about that tomorrow." Tomorrow is a new day. As I was ruminating one evening about this or that problem, the friend I was ranting to gave me some good advice: Things always look better in the morning.

Stop it! Pick up your thoughts about food again in the morning. The sunrise brings a new day. Guilt needs to be put to bed, never to rise with the sun, say I, who just indulged in six sugar cookies!

The Elephant in the Room—Stress

There are enough "don'ts" in the diet world to give us all a lifetime of heartburn. Some you might have heard are:

- **Don't** eat standing up at the kitchen cupboard because you have to run out the door "five minutes ago."

- **Don't** eat on a TV tray in front of the TV watching a fast-paced James-Bond-style chase scene, as it will result in the fast-paced chugging of food. What happens when we eat too fast? We don't even know we've eaten, as we haven't given our food time to settle, which means we just want to eat more and more.

- **Don't** eat while driving. Reasons for that rule include the safety of yourself and others as well as digestion.

- **Don't** polish off your dinner while texting your friend or while talking on the phone.

- **Don't** eat and run. Eating a meal is not the same as running a marathon.

- **Don't** eat in your car after the carhop brings out those burgers on a tray that she so charmingly attaches to your car window at the A&W Root Beer stand. Oops…that one doesn't exist anymore. In fact, the old A&W stand in my neighborhood was turned into a sushi takeout place.

- **Don't** eat dessert.

- **Don't** eat seconds—or thirds or fourths.

- **Don't** eat carbs.

- **Don't** be a couch potato.

- **Don't** eat too much salt.

- **Don't** drink soda pop.

Let's see, what did we do right in the convent? We ate at the table in the dining room. We all ate together. No one ate in the recliner in front of the TV, no one bolted down food to run to a ballgame, and no one rushed out to a League of Women Voters meeting.

However, we *did* eat dessert, and we did a lot of the other don'ts as well. We are not all going to hell—at least not for these food reasons—and we were not scolded by the mother superior for an occasional snigger during a silent meal.

We all know the don'ts are probably mostly correct but hard to follow. Do the best you can but forget about the rest as a jumble of don'ts. Take one thing at a time.

Think about creating a mealtime atmosphere that allows you to savor your food, enjoy the sights and sounds around you, and if possible, be with the people you love. Even though we did not speak during meals in the convent, there was still the comfort of companionship—and someone with whom to share a stifled giggle if something went awry during the meal.

My widowed mother, who ate alone most of the time, liked to light a candle and listen to a country music CD while she ate. As an adult, I have lived alone most of my life and liked to do the same—though it wasn't always country music. Now I enjoy dining with my husband, sharing events of the day. Create a family dining tradition that works for you. But remember the adage: After me you come first. Maybe this isn't about fixing the family routine but about fixing it so that whatever *you* need works for you.

STRESS AND WEIGHT GAIN

There's an old saying: "How do you eat an elephant? One bite at a time." Yet it's hard to "eat one bite at a time" or take one step at a time if we don't know what we're eating or where we're stepping. Whether it's a weight-maintenance plan or a financial plan, the approach is the same: We need to start *now*, one bite at a time. Before you can create your plan following the Seven Holy Habits, you have to face the elephant in the room called stress.

Let's take another bite out of that elephant in the room.

Stress is that invisible, heavy cloak we all wear. It's the elephant in the room that keeps us overwhelmed and frozen in our tracks. Stress will always be with us. We need to learn how to live with it and even harness its power to work in our favor.

Stress is an intangible thing, and weight loss is very tangible. How many of us reach for that Nestlé Crunch bar while working at our desk to meet a deadline? How many of us snack continuously after dinner while watching TV out of boredom or to "relax" and relieve the stress of the day? More important, how many of us do these things as a lifestyle because we are living a lifestyle of stress?

We see the pounds adding up on the scale, if we dare get on the scale, or if we even have a scale in the house! We don't want to know....Is it possible to lose weight while under stress? Do we give up because our lives seem to be continuously stressful and we don't see a way to change our lives?

It takes strength, mindfulness, courage, and support from friends, advisors, and loved ones to make a change. Do we start by saying "I'm going to lose weight now"? Or do we say, "I need to reorder my whole life before I have time to lose weight"? The latter will certainly not work and will only cause delay. The former statement is too broad and lacks specificity.

When I feel like I'm smashed under a brickload of stress, it's hard to start something new or look at the old with gutsy honesty for starters. Do I need to visit the psychiatrist to work through my stress? Perhaps for some people at various times in their lives, that's true. The first bite out of the apple of stress needs to be the question, "Where am I now?" In my work as a Certified Financial Planner, sitting with someone in anticipation of creating a financial plan, I started with the question, "Where are you now?" Then I asked, "Where do you want to go?" This was followed by a discussion of how to get there. That first bite out of the apple of stress is the question, "Where am I now?" and it needs to be spoken out loud. For example: "Where I am now is overweight. Where do I want to go? I want to lose 50 pounds and keep it off forever." And finally, "How will I get there?"—and that is the 64-thousand-dollar question.

Before you can "get there," you need to look at all the things that are in the way. Some of those things have been discussed: lack of good habits (a plan), lack of a routine for following the habits, and lack of willingness to build the habits required (the ability to stick with the plan). Also, lack of tenacity to start over again as many times as it takes to reach the goal. Dealing effectively with stress will free you to accomplish all your goals and get to the finish line.

The title of this book is not *How to Manage Stress*, and I'm neither a doctor nor a therapist, so I can talk only about my own experience and what works and has worked for me.

As a financial planner meeting with clients, I would often hear things like, "I guess that really wasn't a wise investment choice I made in the past," or "I should have saved and invested more"—or "at all." My answer to all such questions was always, "You *did* make the right choices, because you took action and did *something*." Or, if nothing had been saved to date, I would say, "You're here now to begin, so you *have* taken action." Don't let the negative stress of past actions or lack thereof hamper you in the future. Today is the first day of the rest of your life, as the saying goes. Let that heavy cloak of negative stress fall away, and begin anew. Just know that every new day will bring with it stress. It's how you handle that stress that matters. Can you harness it as new energy to propel you forward?

Being afraid of making the wrong decision often causes people to make no decision, which will inherently be the wrong decision. No decision is a decision made by others or by circumstances. You no longer own your own destiny. Make a decision in order to begin. If you begin on the wrong path, as seen in hindsight, you can always make a course correction. Fear of making the wrong decision is its own stress and brings about inertia and procrastination, also major causes for stress. This mental process will keep you running like a rat in a maze, chasing your tail.

Maybe weight gain is causing the stress? It's like, which came first, the chicken or the egg? The stress or the weight gain? Who cares? Jump on the carousel and start moving even if it feels like you are only moving in circles!

Make a plan and work your plan...action, action, action. The Seven Holy Habits are just ahead, waiting to help you make that plan and take action.

For me it's helpful to think back on periods of my life during which I did not feel more than normal stress and I was able to maintain my weight easily. The first of those takes me back to my days in the convent. Did I experience stress in the convent? Yes. There is good stress and bad stress, short-term stress and long-term stress. Without some sort of stress to push us, we would probably do nothing but sit in front of the TV all day eating bonbons. Yes, there was stress in the convent, but on balance the stress led to positive actions and feelings of peace and accomplishment. During that time, I lost 50 pounds.

Every morning there was the stress of getting dressed: Would I be able to pin on the headpiece of the habit straight without a mirror? Would I do it in time to make it to morning prayers without being late? That was a type of stress quickly forgotten after I slid into the chapel pew on time most mornings. There was also the stress of looking around to see who was missing. In those days, over 50 years ago, when a girl decided to leave the convent, it seemed to happen in secrecy. Nothing was said. We knew someone had left by her absence. Depending on who was missing, the stress was more or less great. Was it a friend I had bonded with, or was it someone I really didn't know? There was some feeling of sadness or emptiness in not having been able to say goodbye. Again, this is an example of a short-lived stress quickly swept away by the day's routine, new discoveries, and new friends.

There are certainly greater stresses in life than those listed above. Stresses that we must learn to live with or change if we can, having the wisdom to know the difference between the two, as goes the "Prayer of St. Francis" hanging on my bedroom wall. Such stresses include: sickness, death, job loss, not enough money to pay the bills, a wayward child, you name it.

Ongoing and serious stress is often best dealt with "the convent way" for me: prayer and meditation, advice from various professionals and loved ones, and action where possible, or effective acceptance when action won't work.

I find that creating and sticking to a good schedule and good habits on a daily basis brings peace and accomplishment. Good habits help me resist the urge to snack. A good schedule has some yummy snacks built into it, because I know I can never go a lifetime without a snack.

Interruptions bring chaos and frustration. Convent life was so lovely without all the interruptions of secular life. I forever look to cleanse my life of interruptions and accept those that can't be helped, ordering them under my control as much as possible. A certain acceptance of ordered interruptions will help bring peace to chaos.

A sense of accomplishment is also a stress reliever. In the convent, successfully completing each day was its own accomplishment. A meal artfully prepared in Priests' Kitchen, a cutwork tablecloth beautifully ironed, or a difficult passage in Beethoven's "Moonlight" Sonata practiced and conquered at the piano brought with it a sense of accomplishment, just one day and one bite at a time. Underlying these accomplishments were the morning prayers, the Mass with its beautiful hymns, the spiritual readings during meals, and the prayers at night. How can I order my days as a layperson in this way? The answer to this question doesn't require 1) a comprehensive financial plan for life, 2) the instant loss of those extra eight pounds, 3) walking the Derby Day 5K, or 4) a return to the monastery.

Address the elements of everyday life on all fronts. For example, "Today I will do the following: 1) get all the house bills in one folder, 2) leave the last bite on my plate at breakfast, lunch, and dinner, 3) take a morning or evening 30-minute walk around the neighborhood, and 4) complete one page of spiritual or motivational reading."

Write down these goals and check them off at the end of the day. That feeling of accomplishment will drive the stress away. It doesn't matter if the four things weren't accomplished with perfection. Suppose you couldn't find all the bills and discovered that you were missing one, ate everything on your plate at dinner because you "just couldn't help it, the food was so good," went out to walk but it was so hot you could only manage ten minutes, and you were too tired for spiritual or motivational reading at 10 p.m. so you just said, "Thank you, God, for this day." Tomorrow is a new day; just "carry it forward."

The Seven Holy Habits that follow, as well as the reflections on what I've learned, will provide tips for a more ordered day, for creating a life of your own choosing, and for making food your friend.

PART III

THE SEVEN HOLY HABITS

Visualization: You're Thin Until You're Thin

What on earth does that mean: You're thin until you're thin?

That's Holy Habit #1, Visualization: You're Thin Until You're Thin." Visualization is seeing a picture in your mind's eye. It can be a fantasy or it can be a vision of the future. We might also call this using your imagination. For example, as I shop for a new dress for my five-year-old, I take a dress off the rack and envision my daughter wearing that dress at her birthday party and looking like the prettiest child in the room. Reading a novel is imagining. Childhood play with paper dolls requires imagining stories about each doll.

I imagine what the grounds around the convent will look like when spring comes and everything turns green. This isn't hard to imagine because I've seen such a sight before. Nature takes care of painting the spring green; I don't have to do anything about it.

I also dream of playing the piano again as I once did. I look back.... As I practice Bach's "Chromatic Fantasia and Fugue" on the piano, I see myself performing the piece flawlessly from memory at a recital. I see myself walking on stage, sitting down at the piano bench, lifting my hands over the keyboard, and beginning to play. I breathe a song into the musical phrases of the piece. My fingers move with my every breath, my wrists relaxed but firm. I feel great strength coming from my upper arms down to my wrists. I feel the agility of my fingers clearly and distinctly playing each note and molding them into phrases. I see the notes running through my head, as they are not on paper in front of me. I see the phrase markings and every printed indication of *andante*, *presto*, or *vivace* on the page. I visualize "Chromatic Fantasia and Fugue" throughout my body as I bring the piece to life with the piano as my messenger. I see myself in command of the keyboard.

I feel great strength as I execute the phrases and movements. I can taste the excitement of the piece as I share it with the audience. I try not to worry about hitting a wrong note, because that doesn't really matter. Expression can be completed even with a wrong note. The piece is not about notes. Playing the notes comes from much practice. Playing those notes is now a habit. Because I know the notes, I don't think about the notes. I think about my calling as an artist to bring this great work of Bach to life for my audience. I know if I worry about hitting a wrong note or getting lost in the music that I will do so. I put such thoughts out of my mind as I take the stage to begin my performance. All that matters at this moment is the communication of Bach's "Chromatic Fantasia and Fugue" to my audience. I am merely a conduit; the ego that is "I" is not important. Bach is speaking through me.

As I write this visualization, I feel the excitement I've known, having done in the past what I am now visualizing. I feel energy. I cannot write fast enough. I am sharing on paper a part of my soul as I relive the experience of performing Bach's "Chromatic Fantasia and Fugue." I hear the music now running through my head. I see myself sitting at a shiny black Yamaha concert grand piano. I am excited to have seen the audience as I walked across the stage to the piano bench. I am also very nervous. I am always nervous as I wait in the wings to enter and then cross the stage. I sit down on the piano bench and play the first note and the nerves fall away. The audience no longer exists; it's only about bringing Bach to life with everything in my mind and body. I finish the piece; the applause begins; I stand up and take a bow and walk off the stage. My job is done.

After the concert, I greet the audience members backstage, one by one, as if each person were the only one in attendance at the concert, until I greet the next person and then the process begins again. I hear words of praise and encouragement: "What a fine career you will have as a concert pianist." I am grateful for having had talented artists as piano teachers. I envision graduate school as a piano performance major. With each moment I envision, I am only in that moment. Nothing else matters. The fact that I am a poor sight reader does not matter in this moment. Artists have a talent for visualization, but it is a talent we can all develop. I played the piece as an artist, not as a piano student. I am an artist. I see myself as an artist. As I put pen to paper describing this visualization, the performance experience feels real and current. In fact, the event took place 50 years ago.

Today I visualize that I will again be able to play the piece as I once did. This is a dream. Learning and performing a piano piece does not come around like the green of spring, without work on my part. Only if I practice the piano again regularly can this dream become a reality. I tell myself, "I played this piece once with fine interpretation, and I can do it again."

I dream of playing that Bach "Chromatic Fantasia and Fugue" again, but so far I haven't unpacked the music and started to practice. If I don't find the sheet music, set it on the piano, open the keyboard cover, and start practicing the piece note by note, I will never again play the "Chromatic Fantasia and Fugue." I can listen to a recording of my playing that piece for inspiration, to help me visualize doing it, to remind myself that I did it because it would be me playing on the recording that I would be listening to. Will this drive me to the piano to practice or just make me feel nostalgic and wistful about what was? I am at a crossroads. Am I going to play those notes again and again until they become a habit, so I can work on interpreting the piece?

The same thing is true with weight loss and maintenance. Maybe I used to be thin. Maybe I've dieted before and been thin again for a while. I've dieted before and maybe not been so thin. Maybe I gave up. The negativity of it all just became overwhelming. I lost the vision. The fascinating hook of a new diet will never be motivation enough to keep someone thin for a lifetime. Strong and constant visualization can do the job, however.

This is the same strong visualization that I use to see possibilities, to see realities, in the future, that I've never done. I'm not afraid of hard work. If that's all it takes, I can do it. I dream of being thin. I personally was never thin before I became thin in the convent. Maybe I wasn't too fat until I was about age six. Maybe I was "thinner" the summer before sixth grade because my friend Karen and I went swimming every day. It didn't last. I imagine that I will walk into a room as a thin person and everyone around me will "ooh and aah" and compliment me on my weight loss. I see in my mind's eye a thin person. I visualize that I am thin. I look through fashion catalogues and see a beautiful dress on me instead of on the print model. As a child, I always wanted my mother to order dresses for me from the Montgomery Ward catalogue. She never did, but she never said no. She just said nothing. Later I realized that the standard children's sizes listed wouldn't have fit me. Ordering a dress would only have caused heartbreaking disappointment for her little girl.

Now as an adult I look at the catalogue and see myself in the dress looking the same as the model looks in the dress. It's tempting to order the dress from the catalogue, but I think, "What if the dress makes me look fat and I just have to return it?" I don't order the dress because I don't want to spend hard-earned money only to be disappointed, to have a rude awakening from a delicious fantasy. Do I just close the catalogue and close the door to my dream of wearing that dress and looking like that fashion model, or do I let that catalogue speak to me? While I continue to dream, the catalogue picture becomes part of my vision board. I cut out the picture, stick it on the refrigerator with a magnet. That becomes my vision board. A vision board spurs us to act. I begin speaking the mantra, "I will be thin," first to myself and then out loud. Thinking thin will not remain just a pipe dream. If I say it out loud, I will be accountable to others. I will become thin.

To become that thin person I used to be or that I want to become, I must practice "the notes" so they become a habit. Yes, I lost 50 pounds, but that did not turn me into a fashion model. I am too short, too old, and not thin enough to be a fashion model. I accept my height, age, and weight. Thin for me means being satisfied with a realistic weight I am able to *maintain forever*. I would rather weigh 138 and maintain it than diet down to 128 and start gaining again as soon as I stop dieting. After all, one can only eat "two peas on a white plate" for so long before going back to eating the old way, which may have included eating anything in sight. Maybe my vision board should not have a model from a fashion catalogue pinned to it. Maybe I should pin up an old picture of a thinner me, or of a friend of reasonable weight. I am as tall and as young as I will ever be, and I'm thin enough to feel good about myself. For people who did not know me when I was heavy, the only person they know is a normal-size woman—not too tall, not too short, not too fat, and not too thin.

Once a fat person, always a fat person, in some people's mind's eye. To this day, I look in the mirror and think: I look fat. I haven't looked fat for 50 years. Some clothes make me look thinner than others, however. Choose what makes you look slimmer, what makes you feel good about yourself.

I fight the "I look fat" neurosis and negative self-talk. I look in the mirror again and see a person who looks pretty good. I see a person who is no longer young, a little thick in the middle, but "thin." I'm satisfied with my appearance for the day and dig into focusing on all the other things that really matter in my life. My day cannot be about my weight and negative self-talk and introspection. Years ago, during our convent "formation" period, I learned to feel good about myself, to look outward, to help others. What will your day be about today? Check thoughts about weight at the door, knowing you are putting the weight-loss habits in place. Walk through the door and begin your day.

I don't have to be fat because I can visualize being thin.

I imagine I'm thin until I'm thin. It takes time to lose weight and I don't want to wait, so I put on the head of a thin person.

If I could have the head of a nun and then the head of a musician and then, for 30 years, the head of a financial planner, why not the head of a thin person?

Visualization has been the most important habit of my success. I visualize being thin. If I start to gain weight, I visualize how terrible it felt to be fat. Losing weight and keeping it off start inside. They have everything to do with how I think about myself and how I feel about myself. I have to start here. I was fat beginning at about age six, and it felt terrible. The misery I felt as a fat child and teenager comes to mind if I get off track for some reason and start gaining weight, start getting fat again. Getting off track happens often at times of life changes: getting married, having a baby, going on vacation, having surgery, retiring, and the like. I look in the mirror and see that fat person I used to be, and I pass on the second helping of macaroni and cheese.

Maybe the opposite is true for you. As a young person you were thin, and now you are startled to see a fat person in the mirror today. Visualize how grand it felt to be thin, to be picked by the sixth-grade team captain for the school's baseball team. (The fat kid was the last one chosen.) How did it feel to go out on a date in high school looking thin and lovely? (Fat girls don't generally date.) If you were thin, your father didn't have to pay someone to take you to the prom, an experience that was mine.

Imagine being thin. It doesn't matter whether you've been thin in the past, gained weight and lost it a dozen times before, or never lost the weight at all. Do not be afraid. Actress Faye Dunaway once told *Esquire*, "Fear is a pair of handcuffs on your soul."

Just daydream. What did you do in school when you were sitting in class listening to a boring teacher drone on about the Peloponnesian War between Athens and Sparta in 404 BC? You were daydreaming about meeting friends after school at the drugstore to hang out. I daydreamed about going uptown with my mother, sitting in the hair salon reading a book while she got her hair and nails done, knowing that soon we would be having lunch in the Golden Rule department store's dining room. Maybe there would be a runway fashion show in the dining room. I would revel in one of my favorite combinations: food and fashion. My mother was thin and looked good in every fashion. I watched her and felt proud that I had such a beautiful mother. I tried not to think about what I looked like. A daydream can include recalling a pleasant past event or the vision of a future goal.

We can never be too old or too jaded to dream, to imagine and then turn those dreams and imaginings into the visualization of a goal. If you have lost weight and regained it many times in the past, don't be afraid to try again in a different way. Don't be too discouraged or jaded to try again.

DIFFERENT CAN MAKE A DIFFERENCE

Today is a new day, and what I'm saying here is most likely different than what you've tried before. Sometimes when we hear something said just a little bit differently, the light bulb goes on and a new understanding sets in. Any worthwhile goal is worth returning to and/or continuing the effort to achieve. In the game of losing weight, all approaches are fair and all helpful tips are fair.

Set aside all negativity and despair, and approach losing weight with the openness of a child. If you can daydream, you can imagine, you can visualize, and you can set a goal and begin again or begin for the first time.

1. <u>Enlist the support of those around you: a spouse, child, friend, or mentor.</u> Shout your goal to all who will listen. Saying, "I'm going to lose weight and keep it off" out loud gives you both support and accountability. Your friends and family will cheer you on (support) and ask how many pounds you have lost so far (accountability). This is a very hard thing to do. I never want to say out loud what it is I'm going to accomplish for fear that I will fail. But I breathe deeply, swallow hard, and tell someone—maybe a stranger at first, because then there will be no accountability. I strike up a conversation with the person sitting next to me on an airplane, talk about losing a few pounds, and know that when we deplane we won't see each other again. This can be good practice. I've wanted to write this book for years. I emailed the thought and a prospective book title to a friend, never followed up, and hoped she forgot I ever sent the email. About eight years later I sent the email again. This time I followed up on it and was surprised at the supportive reception I received from my friend. That gave me courage and energy to move forward.

2. <u>Know your body type.</u> There are three body types: ectomorph (distinguished by a lack of much fat or muscle tissue), mesomorph (marked by a well-developed musculature), and endomorph (characterized by

a preponderance of body fat). Which of these three types are you and why does it matter?

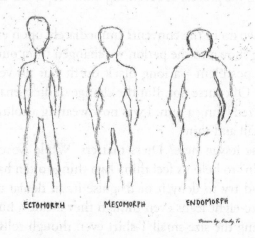

ECTOMORPH   MESOMORPH   ENDOMORPH

Drawn by: Cindy To

Body Types: Ectomorph, Mesomorph, Endomorph

ECTOMORPH

- Narrow hips and clavicle
- Small joints (for example, wrist/ankles)
- Thin build
- Stringy belly muscles
- Long limbs

MESOMORPH

- Wide clavicle
- Narrow waist
- Smaller joints
- Long and round belly muscles

ENDOMORPH

- Blocky
- Thick rib cage
- Bigger joints
- Hips as wide (or wider)than clavicle
- Shorter limbs

3. <u>Dress for your body type.</u> Knowing what to wear will help you visualize being thin. Visualizing being thin and thinking thin are important while you're in the process of becoming thin. Props, like clothes, can help.

What did we do in the convent? Immediately upon entering for the first time and being shown to the parlor, we changed from our street clothes into the habit of a postulant—a long black outfit but no veil. Had I instantly become a nun? Of course not. But the change of dress enabled me to feel like a nun. I visualized being a nun. I was now wearing a column of black, which made me feel tall and thin.

What is the lesson here? Dress matters. While we're losing weight, we must dress "thin" to help us feel thin. Two things often happen when people gain weight and try to deny it or disguise it. In denial mode, we continue wearing our size-eight jeans even though they create a huge muffin top. We continue wearing the size-small T-shirt even though rolls of fat push out in layers around the middle. But we say, "I can still wear a size eight." Really? This is denial. On the flip side, others revert to wearing big blouses and muumuus to hide the weight. Is the weight really hidden, or do we just feel comfortable knowing there's plenty of room for even more weight? If no one can determine visually what's you and what part is just the big blouse, you don't look thin, you look as big as the muumuu.

Let's go back to the convent. We wore black, floor-length, pleated serge skirts. Long and black is slimming. How about a pair of well-fitting black pants? On top, we wore a black cape that grazed over the waist in front, curving upward on the sides, creating the illusion of a waist. How about a top with only a slightly fitted waist, creating the illusion of a waist where perhaps there is only a square block of body under the blouse?

What style of dress is the answer?

- A column of color is always more slimming than two contrasting top and bottom colors. For example, a black blouse and black pants are more slimming than a white shirt with dark pants. Wear a colorful blazer or sweater on top of that column of black.

- Emphasize your best feature: small waist, great legs, well-shaped bust, and so on. Contrast a blousy top with a slim bottom and vice versa. For a thick middle and slim legs, try a blousy top over a slim-cut pant to show off your shapely legs. Tip: Wear your normal size in a blousy top. For a small waist and large hips, wear a shirtdress with a full skirt to emphasize the waist and hide the hips. If you have a thick middle, wear a column of color with a slim belt around the middle to define the waist, and hide the blockishness of the waist with a long cardigan or blazer.

- Jackets can hide a multitude of sins. Wear a longer jacket over a slim bottom and a shorter jacket grazing the top of the hips for a full bottom. Make sure the jacket is not too big and baggy, or it will only make you look thick. A jacket that pulls anywhere or is too small in general will only emphasize extra weight.

- A pencil skirt can be slimming on many people. It can also add the illusion of height. Don't be afraid to try one.

- A long cardigan over pants, a slim dress, or a pencil skirt elongates the body, making you appear thinner.

- Even a low heel worn with pants will make you appear longer and leaner. The most slimming pants style is a straight leg or a boot cut. Don't be afraid to tuck in that blouse. If you feel like a thick or lumpy waist is exposed, top the look with a long cardigan. A blousy top over wide-leg pants will only make you appear heavier.

- *Glamour* magazine suggests flattering features to look for in pants. "For example, flat-front styles. They're instant minimizers if you're curvy. Unlike pleats, a flat front creates an unbroken line across your stomach—making you look taller and slimmer. Also consider a waistband between one and two inches wide. Narrower ones can divide (and draw attention to) a tummy bulge. Pants with a slight flare have long been a top seller for a reason: They make hips look slimmer. And a smidge of stretch helps pants hold on to the clean, sharp fit you bought them for."

- Don't be afraid to try belts. Depending on your shape, a belt sitting on the hip at an angle can be slimming. Sometimes a slightly wider belt can also be slimming.

- Try a wide collar. On a coat, for example, it can be slimming if you are not too short. A long scarf over your usual jacket can also have a slimming effect.

- If you are going to wear separates in contrasting colors, be sure your top does not end at the waist. A more slimming effect is created by having the top end somewhere below your waist.

- Prints can sometimes make you appear heavier than solid colors, depending on the style. Rule of thumb: The smaller the print, the thinner you will look. Often a small-print dress with a self-belt can be slimming when a hip-grazing open jacket is worn over the dress. The self-belt helps define the waist and make it appear smaller—just don't take off the jacket!

- Everyday staple: a pair of straight-leg jeans, a dark top (make sure it ends below the waist), and a long, colorful scarf.

Visualizing keeps us young. Children are not afraid to imagine. Find the child in you and remember, "You are thin until you are thin."

Always Eat Dessert

"Always eat dessert" sounds like something not to do when trying to lose weight or maintain that hard-won weight loss. Yet eating dessert is the very thing that can help keep the weight off for a lifetime as well as help you lose it in the first place. If you enjoy sweets, always eat dessert. (If you suffer from heart disease, are diabetic, or have other health issues and are planning to eat a dessert containing sugar, check with your healthcare provider first.)

How can that be, you may ask? Dessert doesn't have to mean a whole box of Thin Mint Girl Scout cookies or half of a Marie Callender's chocolate cream pie, though many of us understand that dessert language! Dessert *does* mean eating something you enjoy and look forward to eating. If you're gluten-intolerant, maybe dessert means a large gluten-free chocolate chip cookie. If you follow the West Coast juicing and veggie program, maybe it means frozen yogurt topped with strawberries. New Yorkers love their street food, so how about nibbling on glazed apricots from Zabar's while walking down Broadway after dinner? If you're a born-and-bred Midwesterner like I am, dessert means a slice of homemade cake or pie.

You may not be a person who craves sweets, but if that's the case, you probably aren't a person who has a weight problem. In the convent, as mentioned, we always had dessert of some sort. However, it wasn't often a large, fattening dessert, like chocolate fudge cake à la mode. It may have been a small square of a single-layer spice cake with a dab of frosting. However, the apple pie stands out as a premier dessert in my day at Mount Carmel. We had an apple orchard on the grounds.

As noon was the main meal, I remember sitting in daily instruction sessions in the novice community room, with novice mistress Sister Geraldine up in front meting out various life and religious principles, and being distracted by the sweet smell of apple pies baking, wafting up through the floorboards from the bakery below.

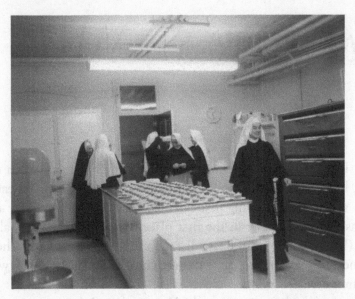

Novices working at bake house duty. It took a team to make that luscious apple pie and those yummy sweet rolls for the approximately 150–175 postulants, novices and professed sisters living in the convent.

We had a lot of apples and ate them six ways from Sunday when in season. The apple pie was the best. Sister Amelia in the bakehouse really knew how to whip up those pies with the help of whichever novice at the time had bakery duty. The pie was served with a slice of cheddar cheese on top, something I had never had and something I didn't think sounded too appetizing. I had never been fond of cheese anyway. But I learned to love apple pie with cheese primarily because the cheese was one more bit of filling food, and I was always hungry. To this day I enjoy a slice of cheese on apple pie. My husband likes it that way even more than I do. (Can my husband's love of the cheese on top of apple pie be explained by saying he is Italian?) An occasional slice of apple pie, with or without cheese or ice cream or whipped cream, isn't going to make anyone fat.

In fact, *here is a secret*, counter to what's said in most diet books, which has been one of the keys to my staying thin for 50 years: *Eat dessert*! Dessert is very satisfying and feels indulgent and forbidden. We always want what we shouldn't have…and a wicked indulgence is very satisfying.

The reason why eating dessert works is because eating sweets signals the end of the meal. After you eat dessert, do you want that second serving of meat and potatoes? Probably not. It's easy to skip seconds on the entrée if you know you can head right to the dessert. And after dessert, who wants seconds?

There were thin girls and there were picky eaters, and both types were good for me to get seconds. The thin girls just filled up on homemade bread, as the bread arrived stacked high on the platter. (Such thin girls sometimes became chubby.) The picky eaters remained thin, it seemed to me, and I got to eat what they picked over. I thought the food in the convent tasted pretty good, and there was a lot of variety. At home, the "family steak" usually resembled brown shoe leather, the potatoes could have passed for hockey pucks, and the canned vegetables arrived at the table dead in the water. I'll take convent casserole—"hot dish," as we call it in Garrison Keeler speak—any day.

The important thing about eating dessert is to make it a guilt-free experience. It is not about being a member of the clean-plate club, and it is not about finishing all the food the kids didn't eat because there are starving babies in Botswana. Eating dessert should be a way of life. Dessert is something to look forward to and enjoy. Spring for a really good dessert. Don't mindlessly finish off a box of bargain-basement sandwich cookies just because they are sitting in the kitchen cupboard. A tip that works for many people, though not for me, is to eat the dessert slowly, savoring every morsel. Try it. This approach may work for you.

In the beginning, it will be tempting to eat too much dessert. People say to me all the time that they can't touch a piece of cake because they won't be able to stop and will end up eating the whole cake. If that happens when you first try the Convent Diet, *then so be it. There's always tomorrow.* The important thing is not to feel guilty, ashamed, weak-willed, or like a failure. Eating too many cookies happens to almost everybody. Welcome to the human race.

This brings me to a very important point that will help when you are tempted to eat the whole cake. *Don't eat dessert alone*, unless of course you live alone, as I did for most of my adult life. If you live alone, the freezer is your friend. Cut that peach pie into five slices (eight slices once you are used to eating less) and put four of them in the freezer. Fruit pie, for example, doesn't thaw in the microwave all that well. If you are tempted to hurry up and thaw a second piece of pie, think about the resulting soggy crust and it will give you pause. If you are really desperate, eat the second piece of pie and notice the watery flavor and texture and remember this the next time you want that second piece of pie.

If you don't live alone, be sure you enjoy your dessert in the presence of a spouse, friend, child, or whoever lives with you. How many of us eat two or three cookies in public and then go home and eat ten or 20 more cookies? We think that is "okay" because no one is looking. Do we really think that? Of course not. That's why we feel guilty after eating the 20 cookies. From now on, eat however many cookies you are going to eat in the company of your spouse and the like. If you are overweight and eat only two or three cookies in the presence of your spouse, that person *knows* you are eating more cookies when he or she is not looking. Your family loves you the way you are now. But your family also will probably want to support you in your efforts to lose weight and keep it off forever. Ask for their help. You will find that you will begin to eat fewer cookies and smaller desserts in the presence of others. Eat what you like so you *stop* the secret-dessert-eating pattern.

In the beginning, give yourself permission to eat "too many" cookies. The Convent Diet does not include any servings of guilt. After all, your loved ones have given you tacit permission to eat too many cookies all along because they love you the way you are. The problem here is generally not those around us. The problem comes from within ourselves. I found the convent to be a very freeing experience. I was accepted the way I was, which provided an encouraging environment in which to grow and improve. I improved intellectually, spiritually, and physically within the environment of community. You can do this too without entering the convent. Your family is your community. Again, if you live alone, create your own community. I lived alone as an adult for about 35 years. I reached out and created a family of friends, associates, and clients—young and old, men and women. I always had people on my Christmas card list. Create your "Christmas card" list and build your community. I learned the importance of community in the convent. Convent life was, at its core, community life.

However, the Convent Diet is not magic. This is where building the crucial habit, Always Eat Dessert, really begins. A habit must be created. Habits are not developed without effort, but that effort will pay off for a lifetime. The old saying, "No pain, no gain" fits here. Studies show that it takes two weeks to six months to develop a habit. I would say you should plan to spend at least six months developing the habit. But what is six months compared with, in my case, 50 years? Healthy habits are holy habits.

In order to be successful, to persevere to the end in creating a habit, you need to be rewarded along the way. Luckily, with the Convent Diet, dessert is its own reward. But in the beginning, that isn't enough. Maybe an old habit needs to be replaced by a new habit? If I have a habit of secretly eating a whole box of cookies before bed, what new habit can replace that old one? Old habits die hard. This is where everyone is different. For example, some people quit smoking cold turkey. Others gradually cut back on smoking, and still others use a medication along with behavior modification to stop smoking.

Food in general, and dessert specifically, is an addiction for some people. Perhaps you are a cold-turkey person and can go from eating a box of cookies at bedtime to eating none. Great. I can't do that. Is it possible to cut back gradually? Are you the kind of person who can cut back from a box of cookies to three-quarters of a box and so on? Do you feel full eating half a box of cookies when you're used to eating a whole box? Drinking a glass of water before tackling the box of cookies can help make you feel full so that fewer cookies are as satisfying as a whole box of cookies. Maybe the habit you need to create here is one of always drinking a glass of water before eating dessert. And if you are truly a dessert addict, perhaps none of these measures will work without professional intervention and/or medication. Only you and your doctor can make that determination.

Take a moment here to stop reading and think about what might work for you to create the habit Always Eat Dessert in moderation. How can you reward yourself? What rewards will it take to rid yourself of all the guilt surrounding this issue? Guilt has to go in the trash for the habit to be honestly created.

There are many ways to free yourself from guilt. Maybe loved ones around you could say it's okay. Maybe falling off the wagon is okay. Let's say after five days of eating only a half box of cookies before bed, I go back to eating a whole box. What can happen here? Negative self-talk comes into play and I say, "I can't do this so I might as well forget the whole thing. I'll just be overweight."

The key here is to put this little imperfection in the past. Tomorrow is a new day. Train your brain! Do better tomorrow. The more we don't think about yesterday, good or bad, the closer we get to creating that good habit. Even after the habit is well-formed, we will occasionally fail. When I have an especially good dessert hanging around the cupboard, I sometimes eat more of it even before I get it into the freezer. That happens. This cannot inspire guilt.

We know it is okay to overindulge because tomorrow is a new day and what happened yesterday no longer counts. Many of my Protestant friends say that we Catholics are lucky because we have confession. We go to confession, confess our sins, do our penance, and start over with a clean slate and no guilt. This is exactly the mind-set needed to create a good habit. Once the sun rises on a new day, yesterday doesn't count. Focus on today's new schedule and all the wonderful things you will experience and accomplish. Forget about anything negative, like eating too many cookies, and focus on moving forward. That's what we did in the convent. The new day called us to do new things and think new thoughts. We did not live in the past; at least we tried not to.

There is, even at this point of our discussion, an elephant in the room. What if my goal is to lose 20 pounds in time for my daughter's wedding next month? The Convent Diet isn't going to solve this problem. Quick-fix diets never allow one to develop a habit. That's not to say that there never is a time or place for a quick fix. We need to stop here and recognize the difference between a diet and a weight-loss lifestyle. If you need to drop a few pounds quickly, then do it *and don't feel guilty about doing it*. When the wedding is over, return to the Convent Diet and work on developing the lifetime habit while celebrating the weight loss already accomplished.

Let's talk more about the rewards. Did you think of some rewards that would be meaningful to you? For me, rewards are about clothes and fashion. My mother raised me to be a clotheshorse, and I continue with that habit to this day. More dessert can't be the reward for eating less dessert. Food in general cannot be a reward. This may be a habit that needs to be replaced with something else.

I tried an experiment with my cat, Kloe. Kloe usually sleeps on his perch in my office while I write. Periodically he gets up and tugs lightly on my arm to get me to stop typing and pay attention to him, to get up and feed him. If tugging on my arm doesn't work, he never proceeds to clawing my arm. He starts meowing for food. Recently I got up at one of these points, but instead of giving Kloe treats, I got out the laser light that he loves and chased him around the house with it. I chased him until he was worn out from jumping up the wall to catch the laser light. I got a bit of exercise too, by the way, and a break from being glued to my desk chair. Kloe then lay down and went back to sleep. He forgot about begging for food.

When I start trying on clothes and putting new outfits together by "shopping" in my closet, hours can pass by. At the end of the process, I really don't want to eat anything, because the desire to look good in my clothes is more powerful than the craving for a cookie. That's just my story. Perhaps it reveals a certain shallowness, but that's my truth. What is your truth? What is your reward? Maybe your reward is playing a mindless video game; maybe it's calling, emailing, or texting a friend. Your reward has to be something you love, something that makes you feel connected and satisfied, and something that won't make you feel guilty. Perhaps you have two or three favorite rewards—some quick, like stretching, and some a bit more time-consuming, like putting a coat of glitter on your fingernails. Make it a habit to go to those rewards instead of reaching for the extra cookies. In time, two or three cookies will become your habit, not a box or half a box of cookies.

Research shows that up to 90 percent of our food decisions are habits, which saves brain energy for more difficult decisions. If you can make the Seven Holy Habits in this book personal habits, then your life will be free to concentrate on what really matters. In the beginning, energy and focus are needed to create the habit, which then goes on autopilot for a lifetime.

SCIENCE BEHIND THE ALWAYS EAT DESSERT HABIT

Doctor Aaron Beck in the 1960s developed cognitive behavioral therapy (CBT), a psychotherapy that helps people change their unhelpful thinking and behavior. Along those lines, his Beck Institute (just outside Philadelphia) has published articles on the importance of eating dessert for lifetime weight maintenance. To quote Doctor Beck: "We believe that eating dessert, and for many dieters (ourselves included) eating a reasonable portion of dessert *every day*, is an important part of lifetime weight loss and maintenance.... Cutting a food out entirely almost always leads to eventually eating way too much of it....Being overly restrictive just doesn't work long term because it's impossible to stick to forever."

Keeping weight off for 50 years has to be a lifestyle, not a diet. Eating dessert is something most people cannot permanently cut out of their lives.

From a psychotherapy point of view, research also shows that dessert must be enjoyed. While I didn't see any mention of the word "guilt" in my research, I did see explanations of guilt. I did see discussions about the importance of feeling good about eating dessert. When something is forbidden, and we, like Eve, eat the forbidden fruit, we then eat way too much of it. Doctor Beck writes, "It's important not to think that eating dessert means you're offtrack....When desserts are forbidden, getting offtrack will always be appealing."

Eating dessert every day builds in the idea of moderation. A stolen moment eating dessert creates an urgency to eat as much as possible because "I may not get any more again." Because of this urgency, we eat too much dessert. However, if we know we can have dessert again tomorrow...and tomorrow and tomorrow, it takes away the urgency. It's then easier to eat dessert in moderation. In the convent where I'm living now as I write this book, we have homemade cookies almost every night; the flavors vary but eventually always repeat. At first I couldn't get enough of the cookies. Now I know they will be there every night, so I can easily take just one or pass them up completely.

No one is perfect in mastering dessert in moderation. I love rhubarb pie, for example. I no longer buy a whole pie and freeze the slices. Even that approach can be too tempting. In moments of real craving, I don't care how soggy the crust is; I have to have *more*. What I do now is buy one slice and bring it home. That flies in the face of the frugal Midwesterner in me who says a whole pie is cheaper per slice, but the few extra pennies it takes to buy the pie by the slice save my waistline for a lifetime. The lesson here is that you need to find the tricks that work for you to Always Eat Dessert in moderation.

Another thing that works for me: If I've had my dessert and want more, I start darning my socks. (A skill learned in the convent, of course. Go ahead and laugh—I'm just saving the pennies I wasted on buying pie by the slice.) After a while, like my cat, Kloe, I no longer crave more dessert.

Think of eating dessert as your birthright. Enjoy it every day.

Holy Habit #3

Don't Count Calories, But Calories Count

H ave you ever gone on a diet, and you immediately began reading the calorie count on the package of every food item you touched? How long can that last? "I'm supposed to eat 2,600 calories a day; this has 75 calories, so 75 from 2,600 is how much?" Most of us weren't math majors.

Have you ever been on a specialty diet such as a liquid diet, a protein diet, or a cabbage soup diet? Or maybe you've been on a sweets-and-carbs diet. I have learned that selective eating:

- Can result in weight loss (a detox diet, a vegan diet, a protein diet, and so on)

- Can result in weight gain (a fettuccine Alfredo diet, a mac 'n' cheese diet, a fudge cake à la mode diet, and so on)

- Will not result in long-term maintenance of weight loss. Healthy selective eating cannot be maintained for a lifetime, at least not by me. Selectively eating carbs and sweets can and often is maintained for a lifetime, usually resulting in continued weight gain.

Many diets can help you drop a few pounds, or even more than a few pounds, to look better in a party dress for New Year's Eve, for instance, and that's fine in many cases. The Convent Diet is not about losing a few pounds for a short or relatively short period of time.

At the end of the day, if I eat fewer calories, I will lose weight. As my mother said once to my father when he announced for the 100th time that he was going on a diet, "Jim, just eat less." Spoken by a true thin person! Easier said than done.

My convent diet of 50 years ago was essentially the "just eat less" diet prescribed by my mother. In the convent, the calories were counted for us in the form of portion control. We ate whatever the dietitian in the kitchen, Sister Mary Grace Ann, prepared and how much of it she prepared for each of us. During my postulant and novice years, there were probably three-hundred-plus sisters living in the motherhouse at one time, and it was Sister Mary Grace Ann's job to feed us all.

How can you replicate the Convent Diet of old without entering a convent and without feeling deprived? To be blunt, how can you follow the Convent Diet without having the mother superior breathing down your neck, controlling each bite you put into your mouth? How can you "just eat less" on your own, cutting back slowly so as not to feel deprived?

Cutting back on what you eat one bite at a time will result in an "accidental diet." Let's be more specific. If you weigh 200 pounds and should weigh 130, it's going to be different than if you weigh 140 pounds and should weigh 130. If you normally eat two out of three rows of a box of Thin Mints Girl Scout cookies for dessert, for example, start by eating one or two cookies less each night until the new portion becomes satisfying. Leave two cookies in the box at the end of the second row and go watch the news. At the end of the news you'll probably feel full enough.

Continue onward in this fashion until three to five cookies become enough. This will take time. I did not lose 50 pounds in 50 days; I lost 50 pounds in two years. If that's not fast enough for you because your daughter's wedding is six months from now and you want to be thin for it, then use one of the good diets on the market to lose some of the weight faster. Then use the Convent Diet to *keep* the weight off.

It's very difficult to count the calories of every item on the plate at every meal, three meals a day, 21 meals a week, 1,092 meals per year. Our mind would have to be a running encyclopedia of calorie counts. This is not possible for most of us. Another option would be to carry around a dictionary of common foods and their calorie counts—not something I would do.

Like all knowledge, in the beginning it must be acquired. If the information is something we access regularly, calling up that information from our brain file becomes a habit. Sometime around the first grade we learn the alphabet. The alphabet must be memorized. The letters are then applied to words. Soon the knowledge and use of the letters of the alphabet become a habit. We learn more and more words by rearranging, adding, and subtracting letters.

Calorie count is the alphabet we need to make the best food choices. We must learn calorie counts just as we learned the alphabet, and in time calorie counting will become as automatic as reciting the ABCs. The hard part is learning and practicing what you learn on a consistent basis. Learning calorie counts can be done a little at a time, starting with the basics. The basics are simple: What is the calorie content of the foods you like to eat? Don't worry about the number of calories of all the foods in the universe that you might eat.

Make a list of your favorite foods and look up the calorie count for each. This chapter contains a list of many everyday foods and the calorie count for each. The tricky part is knowing the portion size. For example, if one of your favorite entrées is fried chicken and you eat half of a fried chicken for dinner, how many calories have you eaten? Home-prepared fried chicken without a coating may run about 575 calories for a small half chicken. However, half a chicken that is KFC Extra Crispy will run about 1,200 calories. I tend to say to myself: I just ate a half of a fried chicken, without thinking whether it was this or that type of fried chicken. This may be a very unorthodox approach, but I can't keep a lot of food details in my head. So for fried chicken I might just think in round numbers and say to myself: I just ate about 900 calories. I go onward throughout my life thinking of a half of a fried chicken as 900 calories. This thought goes on autopilot and onto the back burner in my mind.

I also know that the best choice of fried chicken for my waistline is not going to be KFC Extra Crispy. If I love KFC and I *really* want fried chicken, not roast chicken, I'll order the KFC Original Recipe as a compromise. Half of an original recipe chicken runs about 400 calories. Another tip: Try to overestimate the calorie count of a food item in your head before you eat it. Doing this makes me feel "safe." This approach is not a typical approach to dieting, but then, I am just sharing with you what I do and how I think, and I'm never on a "diet" anyway.

An average 135-pound woman needs anywhere from about 1,755 calories to 2,210 calories per day *total* to maintain that weight. The variations allow for age, height, and activity level. An older, less active, shorter woman requires fewer calories to maintain 135 pounds than does an active, younger, taller woman. Just one order of half a chicken that's KFC Extra Crispy contains approximately 55 percent to 70 percent of the calories needed for the whole day to maintain the 135-pound weight! I have many short friends who seem to eat much less than I do and don't look any thinner than I do. It's unfair, but life is not fair. In addition, we all have different metabolisms.

I will talk about metabolism briefly in the section on Holy Habit #4, Being a Couch Potato Is Okay, but a thorough discussion of metabolism is a scientific and medical discussion beyond the scope of this book. The internet is filled with information about the subject of metabolism.

If you are reading this section of this book with interest, you probably do not weigh 135 pounds or less. If you weigh approximately 190 pounds, as I did, that requires eating about 5,700 calories per day to maintain that weight. Here's a sample of what I used to eat in one day:

- Breakfast on the go: large blueberry muffin and latte—575 calories

- Lunch: Big Mac, fries, and a shake—1,900 calories

- After-school snack: mixed cold-cuts sub sandwich on a white roll—500 calories

- Dinner: I'll stick to the KFC example of half a fried chicken, extra crispy; mashed potatoes and gravy; mac 'n' cheese; and two biscuits and honey; followed by a slice of Marie Callender's pecan pie—3,444 calories.

The after-dinner snack, eaten while doing my homework, was the real killer. All those As I got in school came at a price. I routinely ate a large bag of potato chips and a 16-ounce container of onion dip for a whopping addition of 1,996 calories.

Day's calorie total: 10,940 calories.

That sounds disgusting! In fact, I often felt disgusted with myself. Another problem for me: All that junk food got expensive. I didn't have takeout food for every meal every day, which is probably why my average daily calorie intake ran closer to the 5,700 calories that supported my weight of 185 to 190 pounds.

We all bring a different food background to the table. If you grew up on a farm, you probably ate lots of fresh vegetables and meat, did chores after school, ran around a lot, and were not fat. Others grew up with an Italian mama who was a great cook, and they ate lots of pasta (my husband, for example). I grew up in a Midwestern small town with a thin mother who was more interested in the League of Women Voters than she was in cooking and food. We thought that all cakes came out of a Betty Crocker box until we ate at a friend's house whose mother served a piece of cake made from scratch.

On the subject of boxed cake mix: In the beginning, it's good to check the calorie count and contents of packaged food as listed on the package. If this is old hat and you know from having been on many diets to read the labels, then maybe now is the time to stop checking the details on the labels. Trust what you know, rely on it, and live your life. You know roughly what's in that cereal that you are about to eat. And maybe you know what a serving size should be as well.

Judging serving size is the hard part. Is half a chicken a serving size? For most people, probably not; it's too much. I, personally, have considered half a chicken a serving for me most of my life. However, as I've gotten older—and shorter—I've found that two or three pieces of chicken are the right entrée size for me now. The starting point to making this Holy Habit #3, Don't Count Calories, But Calories Count, isn't in the details. Don't try to cut back on the food you eat as part of this habit. That's too much multitasking. Just focus on learning the basic calorie counts of the foods you eat and put your brain on autopilot with that information.

An interesting thing will happen. Cutting back on the amount of food you eat will happen as you become aware of just how many calories you are eating. If you're standing in line to order at KFC, and you've learned that half an extra-crispy chicken is 1,200 calories, you may find yourself saying, "What alternative could I order that would still satisfy me and not make me feel deprived?" With this knowledge, I instinctively make better choices and still feel happy and satisfied with the choice I make. Portion control, at least for me, begins to take care of itself when my "back-burner brain" says, "Lots of empty calories in that choice, Mary Lou; how about ordering the original recipe?" Or, if I'm really dying for KFC Extra Crispy, and I've learned that KFC Extra Crispy is more filling because it has all that coating on it, I might order a quarter chicken and end up with about the same calorie content as half a fried chicken with no coating. By having the calorie count of the foods I eat regularly in my head, I automatically make better choices and often order smaller portions *without feeling deprived*. The key here is compromise, compromise, compromise. As a result, you will still feel happy and satisfied without feeling deprived. Compromise is a win-win situation. And doesn't winning mean that we are happy?

To master this habit, remember: Don't Count Calories, But Calories Count. Begin by nailing down the basic calorie count of your favorite foods so you can then forget about counting calories. There is a learning curve to this habit. For me, practicing this habit has been crucial in keeping my weight steady.

In addition to putting your brain on autopilot regarding the calorie count of your favorite foods, which in itself can help you eat less (at least it does for me), here are some other helpful tips for eating fewer calories without counting calories:

- Use a smaller plate; it will look full with smaller portions. You will eat less food and therefore fewer calories. My husband and I often use paper plates to save time on washing dishes, as we both work full-time. I always buy the eight-inch luncheon-size plates, never the dinner size. Buying smaller plates also means getting more plates for the money. That convent vow of poverty apparently hasn't left me.

- Use tall, thin glasses for milk, soda, juice, and the like, and short, wide glasses for water. Now is your chance to think thin! Psychologists tell us that we perceive height more readily than width. For example, we say, "That St. Louis Arch is really tall." Do we ever say, "That St. Louis Arch is really wide?" In fact, the height and width of the arch are the same, I'm told. You will think you're drinking more, and therefore feel more satisfied, drinking juice from a tall, thin, 12-ounce glass than from a short, wide, 12-ounce glass.

- Eat protein for breakfast. Protein makes us feel full longer than anything else. In the convent, we had protein for breakfast every morning, even if on Tuesdays and Thursdays the protein was Spam. You don't have to eat Spam, but eggs are great.

- Eat three meals a day, or more than three smaller meals a day. My husband will say when he comes home after work, "I haven't eaten anything all day. I'm really hungry. How soon will supper be ready?" What he is really saying is, "I want to eat right now, and I have the right to eat everything that isn't nailed down, because I haven't eaten all day." For me, this is like waving a red flag in front of a bull. Whose fault is it that you didn't eat all day, and why does that give you the right to gorge at dinner? In the convent, we had three squares a day like clockwork...not like clockwork, by the clock! Such precision isn't required. This is not a game of golf. But eating three meals a day, or several small meals a day, will keep you from becoming ravenous and overeating.

- As the saying goes, "Out of sight, out of mind." Don't keep that box of cookies around on the kitchen counter. Every time you come to the kitchen, you will see that box of cookies and think it's time for a snack. Snacks are okay. I normally get hungry at about 4 p.m., when my circadian rhythms are low and I feel tired. I know I have more work to do and that dinner won't be until 7 p.m., so I always have a snack around 4 p.m., give or take an hour. My snack is usually yogurt, nuts, trail mix, or a cheese stick. The snack contains protein and often a sweet taste. The protein keeps me going for another two or three hours, and the sweet taste makes me feel satisfied and ready to go back to work right then. I keep the cookies in the freezer and take them out as needed, one or two at a time. Keep snacks for the kids in single-serving packages and believe me, they will know if you snuck one of their snacks. Don't be penny-wise and pound-foolish—literally. Spend a few extra pennies for individually packaged snacks for others, to keep the pounds away from your own middle.

- Don't eat from the package, because you won't realize how much you've eaten. Pour the cheese popcorn out, measured into a bowl. With cheese popcorn having 150 calories per ounce, dig into that bag and pull the popcorn out by the handful, and you will have gobbled up 1,000 calories before you know it. At our house, this is deadly for both my husband and me as we watch the news after dinner.

- Keep the extras in the freezer. I always have some good desserts around, but they are frozen in single servings in the freezer. When I want more than one serving, I am often too lazy to get up, dig in the freezer, find my frozen treat, and microwave it.

- Healthy snacks usually don't come with labels. I've never seen a label on a carrot stick. You get the message.

- Not all fat is bad. Have a little fat with your meal. Fat tells your brain that you are no longer hungry. For example, to my full-fat plain yogurt at breakfast I add not only fruit but also nuts. The fat in the yogurt and the nuts satisfies me and makes me feel full. When I leave off the nuts, I always want something more to eat. *All yogurt is crammed with protein, calcium, and probiotics.* Whole-milk yogurts tend to have more protein and less sugar than the low-fat versions. Be careful, though, about flavored yogurts, which can contain as much sugar as a Snickers bar.

- For dinner, I almost always have a big salad, but I generally don't use low-fat salad dressing. The fat in the dressing is very satisfying. I just don't use a whole lot of dressing.

- Serve yourself; you will take less. Tell yourself there's more on the stove if you want to get up and get it. And, of course, try to switch to the dessert instead of going back for seconds. My husband does not serve himself. If I cook something he really likes, he always wants a huge portion. I coax him into accepting a smaller serving by saying, "There's more if you want it." He almost never wants it.

Just keep in mind that Rome wasn't built in a day. Use this chapter as a reference guide once you have read it. The lists and tips contained here will help keep you on track daily, yearly, and forever. This is a piece of the blueprint I use to stay thin day by day. Somehow 50 years have passed and I'm still relatively thin.

"This is *now*." As the saying goes, this is the first day of the rest of your life. Whatever food habits you developed growing up do not matter. The way you were raised/allowed to eat may be the *reason* you are overweight, but it is not an *excuse* for being overweight for the rest of your life. At some point, you have to take responsibility for your own destiny. I repeat here in another context something my youngest and very successful brother, David, always says, "Whiners never win and winners never whine."

CALORIES PER AVERAGE (NOT DIET) PORTION OF BASIC FOODS

This chart is organized into the following food groups: meat and fish; eggs and cheese; vegetables and starches, including grains; sweets; and

dairy. In each section are listed common foods with a common portion easily cut in half or doubled, and its preparation style, with the calories in round numbers. For example, half of a baked, broiled, or roasted chicken is 600 calories. This could easily be a quarter of a chicken, at 300 calories, or a whole chicken, at 1,200 calories. If the calorie count of an item is slightly over a major number, such as 116 calories, I just think 100; if slightly under a major number, such as 180 calories, I think 200 calories. It all comes out in the wash. I have developed a general feel for the calories of the basic things I eat. I don't get into details. Counting calories one by one won't work for a lifetime. Make your own list of foods you like and develop a chart like this one for yourself.

MEAT and FISH
Half chicken, baked	600
Hamburger patty, ¼ lb.	175
Hamburger with bun	250
Pork chop, 1½ in. thick, about 10 oz., baked	400
2 lamb chops, baked	450
Prime rib, 8 oz.	600
Sirloin steak, 8 oz.	450
Salmon, 3 oz., baked	150
Ahi tuna steak, 5 oz.	150
Cod, 5 oz.	100
Ham steak, 5 oz.	200

EGGS and CHEESE
1 large boiled egg	75
1 slice of basic sandwich cheese (cheddar, Swiss, and the like)	45
3 scrambled eggs	250
Brie cheese, 1 oz.	100
Mac 'n' cheese, 1 cup	300

I always think "50 calories" when I'm taking a slice of cheese, and know deep down if I use a richer cheese, such as Havarti, it will be more like 90 calories.

VEGETABLES and STARCHES
(all veggie calorie counts include a pat of butter)

Green beans, 1 cup	100
Corn, 1 cup	100
Peas, ½ cup	100-plus
Carrots, 1 cup	100
Broccoli, 1 cup	75
Cauliflower, 1 cup	60
Potatoes, boiled, mashed, or baked, 1 cup	100
Potatoes boiled, mashed, or baked, 1 cup with cream	200
White rice, 1 cup, cooked	200
Brown rice, 1 cup, cooked	200
Pasta, 3 cups, cooked	600
White or wheat bread, 1 large slice or 1 medium roll	100
Restaurant-sized bagel	300

SWEETS
(these are killers but I can't live without them, so I don't)

1 slice of chocolate layer cake (□ of a cake), frosted	500
1 slice of fruit pie or 1 slice cream pie (about □ of a pie)	400
1 good-size brownie (not mini, not gigantic)	150
1 good-size chocolate chip cookie (not mini, not gigantic)	100
1 slice of pound cake, 3 oz.	300
1 large square of coffee cake	400
1 big scoop of chocolate ice cream	150
1 scoop of vanilla ice cream	145
1 Hershey's chocolate bar	200
Jelly candy, gumdrops, and so on, 1 cup (my favorite)	150
Dove chocolate square	40
1 cake-style donut	150
1 glazed donut	250
1 medium muffin	300

For restaurant pie, add about two hundred more calories. I love pound cake but don't eat much of it because it doesn't fill me up enough. I love glazed donuts, but if I can choose cake-style donuts without dying, I do so. Muffins are high in calories, so I choose other things.

DAIRY

I don't like milk, so use it only on cereal. I add a quick pour of half-and-half to the cereal to change the taste of the milk. I learned to eat cheese in the convent; before that I wouldn't touch it. If you are a big dairy fan, you may want to develop your own chart for this category.

Milk, 2%, 8 oz.	126
Yogurt, full-fat Greek, 8 oz.	130

We did not have yogurt in the convent. 50 years ago, yogurt wasn't really marketed in this country. I just love full-fat Greek yogurt with fresh berries, sometimes with a drop of honey if I haven't been eating too heavily previously. I often add nuts, maybe five walnuts or pecans chopped, as that little extra fat is very satisfying and takes away cravings. I also indulge in frozen yogurt and eat it often.

Being a Couch Potato Is Okay

D id we go to the gym in the convent? No. Just the thought of having a gym in a convent makes me laugh. I don't think the vow of poverty would allow for treadmills and bicep-curl machines, at least not in my day. However, the convent was built on lots of land. Instead of doing meditation while kneeling in the chapel, many of us did it by going for a stroll down the pine walk. I think the novice mistress felt it was better for us to walk outside for half an hour at 6 a.m. than to sleep in the chapel. I have to admit that I sometimes did my meditation in a vacant classroom, with my head down on a desk, sleeping. If any professed sisters patrolled the halls during meditation and saw me, I never knew it. I was too tired to walk outside, much less pray in the chapel.

We also enjoyed recreation after dinner. Sometimes I missed that activity too because I was still busy doing dishes in Priests' Kitchen. Doing dishes in Priests' Kitchen was its own kind of exercise. Trying to figure out how to get Sister Mary Teresian to laugh took a lot of energy and, I'm sure, calories. Recreation was often playing ball outside or bowling down at the barn.

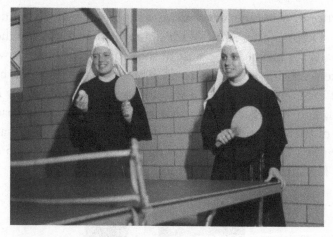

Novices playing ping pong at the barn during recreation. The bowling alley was upstairs.

Some things were fun; others not so much. I wasn't too crazy about our hiking trips led by postulant mistress Sister Anne Marie. Sister was a real mountain goat, leading us up and down the hills, through the brambles and the bushes in long, black outfits on humid, Midwestern, 85-degree days.

There was also plenty of time to sit and read and darn socks; in other words, plenty of couch potato time.

That's Holy Habit # 4, Being a Couch Potato is Okay. It's okay to be a couch potato a lot of the time, or sit and work at a desk much of the day like I do now, as long as you still find time to do something fun and physical. There are 24 hours in a day, and if we spend even one of those hours at a dance class, for example, doesn't that leave 23 hours to sleep and/or be a couch potato? Even better, take a couch potato break during the 23 hours you're not doing something fun and physical and get up and look out the window, step outside in good weather, visit the water cooler, chase the baby, or check on those tomatoes growing in the garden. Make "unconscious" moves like these throughout the day. New research shows that even while you're working at the desk all day it's best to get up and stretch regularly. You're not shirking your office work by getting up and moving; you are improving your work performance and efficiency for your employer, and you're giving yourself a fun break and the gift of a healthy life. I really dislike exercise. You wouldn't catch me dead with a gym membership! However, I just signed up for a clogging class. (Clogging is a type of dance using shoes with taps; it originated in Appalachia.) I love to dance. I show up once a week for the clogging class. I never practice in between classes, as we're supposed to do, but I don't worry about that. Despite Sister Anne Marie's mountain goat hikes in the convent, I love to walk. Or maybe it's because of those hikes that I love to walk. What I didn't like was being out in head-to-toe black clothes on a hot, humid day. After I left the convent, I joined a walking group to raise money for a heart association, and have been doing that ever since. I love the coaches, have made lots of friends, have raised a good amount of money, and as a bonus, have gotten in a little exercise. I'm doing what I love, and I keep moving so that when I'm sitting around I don't feel guilty.

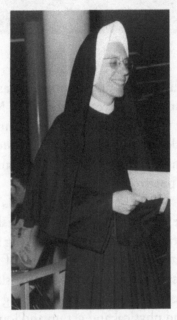

Sister Anne Marie, our "mountain goat climbing" postulant mistress

Here's the key to eliminating exercise, and the accompanying guilt about not doing it, from your life forever: Do something you love that gets you moving. The couch-potato theory of exercise is all about focus. What are some of the things you have done without fail throughout your life because you love to do them and/or you enjoy the people with whom you do them? If you love to play golf, no matter how busy your workload, you will find the time to play golf. As Sister Mary John Thomas said to me in my freshman year of high school, "We always find the time to do the things we really want to do." How many of us can do for a lifetime just the things we *should* do? I *should* visit my mother-in-law, who always criticizes me. I *should* clean out the attic. I *should* exercise. As another friend from my set who is still a nun, Kathy, said to me recently: "There are no 'shoulds' around here." If the "shoulds" in our lives are not things we enjoy, don't we follow the big fat rule of *procrastination*?

I have spent over 30 years as a financial planner. Most people would like to save money and live by a financial plan. Most people do not save money or live by a financial plan. We say to ourselves: "It's August, time to prepare the kids for a new school year, buy the pencils, the erasers, the lunch buckets, and new school clothes. I have neither the time nor the money to save and plan now." Soon it's November: "The kids are in school but now it's time to prepare for the holidays, buy and cook the Thanksgiving turkey, and oh my God, the Christmas/Hanukkah gifts and parties. I have no time or money to plan and save now....When the holidays are over, I'll begin." When the holidays are over and we're settling into the new year, it's time to get paperwork together to do taxes, as April 15 looms large. "Oh my God, I'm going to have to pay extra taxes, so I can't possibly save or plan now." April 15 passes with relief, and pretty soon the kids will be out of school.

Now it's time to plan and budget for the summer vacation. "Hmmm, shall we drive to Niagara Falls and camp, or should we head up to Canada and canoe? I can't do any saving or financial planning right now." We get back from vacation and guess what? It's August again, time to buy the pencils, the erasers, the lunch buckets, and a new year starts in again.

No one wants to visit the financial planner any more than anyone wants to visit the accountant or the dentist. Most of us eventually manage to save a few pennies, face up to doing our taxes, and get our teeth cleaned. Do we do these things like clockwork as often as we should? Probably not, because no one wants to do them. No one wants to diet and exercise either. I shouldn't say "no one." I had a friend and trainer once who seemed to really love to exercise. While she has remained a friend forever, she remained my trainer for about five minutes. I dreaded my sessions with Michelle, and I even had to pay her money to be miserable. That ended quickly. This is not to say that trainers don't help a great number of people; they do. Just not me.

Being serious for a moment, I must say that exercise, that dreaded concept, is good for us; but then so is castor oil. For me exercise and castor oil share the same flavor: terrible.

Can you lose weight without exercising? Of course. An hour at the gym will guarantee nothing for sure in terms of weight loss. (Too many variables for this book or for my expertise.) For some people, exercise increases the appetite. So now the rest of you who have never thought of this have a good excuse for not exercising: It might increase your appetite. However, exercise is good for overall health and for warding off disease, as many in the medical professions tell us. Skipping the after-lunch candy bar will yield pounds lost, all else being equal. For most people, an hour at the gym probably burns fewer calories than skipping the candy bar. During lunch hour at work, would you rather hurry off to the gym, change clothes, hop on the treadmill long enough to break a sweat, take a shower to wash away the sweat, layer on the suit and nylons again, drive back to the office, and settle down at your desk starving because you missed lunch; or just eat lunch minus the candy bar?

Another option: Skip lunch out at the local burger joint; brown-bag it so there's still time to go out for a brief and leisurely walk, sharing stories of the day with friends. For me this is the best of both worlds. I pack my lunch in the morning with foods I like and can afford so that I can enjoy eating. I still have time left over to chat with friends while "accidentally" walking at the same time.

Review this lunch-hour scenario I just described: Am I focusing on exercise? Am I even focusing on dieting? No. I'm focusing on break time, sharing a few laughs with friends. By the way, I got in a little exercise because I went for a walk while talking. By the way, I ate a lower-fat lunch because I packed it myself with things I love that aren't hamburgers and French fries. I've done this kind of thing for years, following the lunch-walk habit I learned in the convent. This could easily become a lifetime habit, or at least a habit followed during the working years.

One of my best friends throughout life was a stay-at-home mom who raised three beautiful, happy, and well-adjusted children. She and other moms in the neighborhood went out for a walk together after breakfast and after the kids went off to school. I recently moved to a 55-and-older community. Many mornings I leave home early and drive through the community on the way to an appointment. I see multiple groups of seniors out walking and chatting as well as solo seniors running, biking, and so on, because it's what they choose to do. Others show up for the tap-dancing class that meets every Monday, Wednesday, and Friday from 10 a.m. to noon. They're enjoying themselves, doing things they love, and by the way getting in a little of that dreaded word, "exercise."

I don't consider my clogging class exercise. I look forward to attending the class because it's fun. Dancing gets me away from my desk, engages my mind with learning new routines (rather than thinking about financial plans and numbers), and gives me plenty of opportunity to chat with newfound friends while sharing a common interest. Is this a kind of multitasking? I can't type fast enough right now, because I am visualizing being in the clogging class, how much fun it is, and how excited I am to share this story. This is what exercise needs to be in order to be important enough and pleasurable enough to do it for a lifetime.

In 2001, a year during which I had my own financial planning practice, assistant, associates, interns, and lots of overhead in a high-rise building on a main business thoroughfare, I received a flyer in the mail looking for people to run/walk marathons to raise money for the American Stroke Association. I have a brother who was severely disabled at age 35 by strokes. So I announced to everyone in my office after opening the flyer that I was going to train to walk a marathon. I was met with unanimous exclamations that I didn't have time to do that. Of course, they were right. I didn't have time to do that, but I signed up to do that anyway. Training was every Saturday morning at 6:30 a.m., not my favorite hour. Undeterred, I began training. I showed up faithfully and on time. Always the one to multitask, I thought I could get in some reading while I walked. The coach did not look kindly on my seemingly cavalier approach to training. Thus began our cat-and-mouse game. Just because I liked to read and walk didn't mean I was going to cut corners and cheat—take shortcuts—along the route. The coach figured me wrong and tried to catch me taking shortcuts. And so I began as the coach's least favorite trainee. Time passed, and I quit trying to read while walking. Sparring with the coach turned into a long-term friendship.

It was also during this time that I was diagnosed with breast cancer and underwent two lumpectomy surgeries. My surgeon had run six marathons and gave me some good tips for how to do the marathon in my condition. It took me seven hours to complete my first 26.2-mile marathon in Las Vegas, but I crossed the finish line and got my medal.

I continued with the program for the next ten years, raising money and walking marathons at least once a year, sometimes twice a year. (Thank God, at least, that the training start time was changed from 6:30 a.m. to 7 a.m.) I do believe it all started with hikes up and down the hills led by our postulant mistress. I envision Maria von Trapp leading those children over the mountains to safety in *The Sound of Music* when I think back to Sister Anne Marie leading a single file of postulants up and down the hills.

Was it exercise that made me stay with the program of the American Stroke Association (now part of the American Heart Association)? I saw many people come and go thinking that walking a marathon was going to be their magic key to weight loss. I saw many people leave the program in disappointment because they didn't lose significant weight. All that walking *did* keep me healthy and in shape. Maybe I dropped a couple of pounds as well over the years. Did I stay with the program on behalf of my stroke-disabled brother? Not really. I stayed with the program because I looked forward to the Saturday-morning camaraderie and fun.

The warm-up exercises we did in the park before we began our run were okay, because they were short and done with friends. After the exercises, we all started out on the prescribed route, walking the prescribed mileage for that day. Sometimes I walked in a group. Sometimes the coach asked me to walk with someone and share my stories for encouragement, because I had been around so long and knew the ropes. Most of the time I dropped off, walked at my own pace, listened to books on my iPod (no more attempts to read), and checked out the new buds and birds in springtime and the leaves in the fall. I was always pleased with myself when I conquered the back hill in Griffith Park in good time.

After training, I never felt better. It was such a great way to start the weekend. I'd heard of the "runner's high," and I guess that's what I was feeling. Endorphins are released during exercise and other positive activities. Endorphins are natural chemicals in the body that fight pain. At the end of my walks and party time with my team, I felt no pain! Maybe I was addicted to the sensation created by walking those marathons. Maybe a more positive way to say it would be: I created the habit of walking every day. Addictions are associated with negatives. In a way, a habit in this context can be thought of as a positive addiction. The habit has to be something we can't do without. We say, "I'm addicted to chocolate; I'm addicted to ice cream; I'm addicted to potato chips," and in my case I say, "I'm addicted to Nutella." I love Nutella so much, I can't keep it in the house or I'd eat it all up in a day. But I'm also addicted to walking. Walking every day has become a habit.

I walk because I *want* to walk, not because I *should* walk. However, I needed the crutch of raising money for a cause I cared about to get me started. I needed the crutch of friendship to keep me walking. If I ever think about going out the door for a walk because I *should* get some exercise, I would probably quit walking on the spot. I continued to raise money for ten years and am still walking marathons 15 years later. I don't consider walking marathons exercise. I consider it an adventure.

Not everyone will find his or her calling in walking marathons. And while I trained on Saturdays, I generally walked an hour each night during the week. As my office staff said, "You don't have time to do that." I gave it what time I could; I compromised, but I made time for it.

It's so important to find something you love that you can do a little bit of every day, alone or with others, as is your preference. That's the key to feeling justified in being a couch potato. If I spend just an hour a day doing something I enjoy that gets me moving, I won't have to feel guilty about sitting around reading a book, watching the ballgame, or working at my desk the rest of the day. Maybe the hour a day is ten-minute segments of playing with the children, or walking the dog, or riding bikes after work and after school with the kids, my spouse, or a friend. Maybe your get-moving time is chasing your cat around the house with a laser beam. You won't stop doing things like this, because they're necessary for the children, spouse, cat, or dog, and they're fun for you. There's no need, then, to feel guilty about being a couch potato the other 23 hours of the day.

I was talking with a nun over lunch recently about weight loss. Sister was quite a bit overweight, not young, used a walker, and was not in the best of health. Yet she was most emphatic in telling me about the exercises she was supposed to do. I listened carefully and asked, "Do you do these exercises?" Of course, her answer was no. We both laughed. I asked Sister about the kinds of things she liked to do and found out that she loved to play the piano. I asked if she still played the piano. You guessed the answer. It was no. I suggested that Sister stop by the piano after lunch before going back to her room and play for a while. Playing the piano is more exercise than not playing the piano. You may laugh, but having been a piano performance major in college, I know the upper-body strength and deep breathing it takes to play the piano. It's not unlike lifting weights. Can't this be a good way to start?

Seeing life with a positive spin is not being Pollyanna. It starts with positive self-talk and positive self-worth. It begins with self-acceptance. We are who we are and where we are, and we go from there.

Growing up, I spent my childhood saying, "What if?" My "what ifs" tended to be negative. What if the 2-garage being pulled up the hill by the flatbed truck falls off the truck? What if, on the first day of school, no one likes me? What if I can't get all As in school? What if I forget the words to the song while singing a solo? My "what ifs" ranged from things and people around me to myself. The negative "what ifs" about me were simply negative self-talk. Sometimes the negative self-talk came from the outside: "Oh, Mary, you're always eating," or, "Oh, Mary, why do you always look down at your shoes when I introduce you to someone?" If we hear negatives about ourselves growing up, sometimes they become our negative self-talk as an adult. We also internalize negatives even if they don't come from the outside. I said to myself as a child, "I'm not as pretty as Patty Roberts. I don't have blonde curls like Marcia and Melanie Mullen. I'm not thin like most of the other girls in my class. I'm taller than everyone in the class except Robert Cash." Accepting the negatives about myself—I'm too tall, I'm too fat, I'm not pretty, despite a supportive mother's telling me otherwise—only led to more overeating, more negative self-talk, and a greater and greater lack of self-worth.

I tried to compensate by getting straight As in school. Achievement was the only way out. I found two best friends who liked me despite all my self-proclaimed negatives—two best friends who accept me to this day no matter what I do or how many bad decisions I make. I was amazed that these girls genuinely liked me; me, who was so unlikable. All three of us were very idealistic and wanted to be "good" girls. We were inspired by the sisters who taught us in school. I had four years of high school in which to learn and develop a bit of self-confidence, not in my looks but in my abilities and talents. In my all-girl high school, it was okay not to be a beauty.

Positive self-talk is truth, not delusion. It's not being Pollyanna, because it recognizes truth. It's the self-talk that allows me to see walking and tap dancing as fun and not exercise. The self-talk that says, "It's okay to sit on the couch and read a book." The self-talk that says, "It's okay to be a couch potato."

Holy Habit #5

Don't Be on a Diet in a Restaurant

Have you ever gone out to lunch or dinner with friends and upon being seated at the table, menus in hand, one of your friends says, "I'm on a diet, so I have to see if there's anything here I can eat"? Your friend proceeds to order a grilled hamburger patty with grilled tomatoes and cottage cheese—actually not that dietetic but often on the diet section of the menu. Your friend on a diet is either truly a bit pudgy or is a toothpick who can never be too thin. I am the champion of being "average," which means not that thin but not heavy either. If I had to maintain a weight ten pounds less than I weigh, I would have to be on a diet 24/7. I am not a movie star and not in the fashion-model business, so why worry about it?

This is your favorite little Italian neighborhood place and you're thinking, "I can't wait to dig into a big piece of lasagna and lots of Italian bread." The diet announcement by your friend makes you feel guilty to even think about ordering such fattening food. I also have a husband who, the day I decide to go all-out and grill rib-eye steaks with stuffed baked potatoes, comes home and says, "I'm on a diet." In my playbook, diets are not allowed. I'm too polite to say anything, but inside I just simmer. (There are exceptions to this rule, but I will get to them later.)

For most of my life, going out to dinner was a special occasion. I still have that feeling, so I don't want it to be ruined by being on a diet. A weight-maintenance lifestyle should allow for enjoyable dinners out. It's my time to have something I just love that maybe I don't cook at home. I don't want to feel deprived and/or guilty. If you have developed the habit of maintaining your weight, having what you want to eat in a restaurant once in a while won't be a problem. I'm told that it takes three days for beef to pass through the digestive system in terms of the number on the scale, but are three days and

111

the extra calories a big deal in relation to a lifetime? I'm not talking about a diet measured in days, weeks, or even months. I'm talking about a lifetime of weight maintenance. Now that I am older, I notice that it takes a lot longer to recover from a night out of candlelight, checkered tablecloths, wine, and lasagna.

Okay, I savor my lasagna, wine, and bread. When I was younger I could polish off half a loaf of French bread and half a bottle of wine without doing too much damage. That's not so anymore. I try to make do with two pieces of bread and butter, *but* if I'm not successful in that effort, I don't worry about it. I practice a little extra mindfulness of what I eat when I get home.

When it comes to weight maintenance, I have thrown perfection out the window. I'm a nitpicking Virgo, so I have to work at accepting my imperfections. If the portion of lasagna served to me is true restaurant size, I often ask for a box right away and put at least a bit of it in the to-go box. What I don't see, I can't eat, and I quickly forget about it in the presence of a good friend or my dear husband. I draw in the candlelight and atmosphere, which becomes its own portion of food to savor. For this reason, I don't like to eat in short-order restaurants. Such food is invariably very fattening and is eaten quickly in an utter absence of enjoyment and atmosphere. I like to save my pennies, eat out less frequently, and choose casual dining over takeout burgers with chili fries. Junk food on a regular basis will be the death of the Convent Diet weight-loss/maintenance program. An occasional junk food splurge, however, may be exactly what is needed to keep you on a lifetime weight-maintenance plan.

When I recently returned to the convent, three meals a day were served buffet style. I thought I'd died and gone to heaven. There were so many choices, and I didn't have to cook any of it. The dinner the first day included roast pork and beef corned brisket, so I took a full serving of each. I soon learned that there were two entrées daily to provide people with a choice. I had thought it meant that one of everything was the order of the day, especially if I couldn't decide between the two. Sides included au gratin potatoes and macaroni and cheese. I definitely had some of each of those two choices! Then I proceeded to the salad bar....Was I at Sizzler? How could such small bowls fit everything presented at the salad bar? There was fresh spinach, chopped lettuce, and all the usual accoutrements, such as tomatoes, carrots, beets, cucumbers, green onions, sliced onions, shredded cheese, black olives, green olives, and more. Next came a tray of maybe potato salad, tuna salad, egg salad, three-bean salad, two types of Jell-O salad, cheddar cheese cubes, and finally seeds and croutons for toppers. In this group, I went for the greens and skipped the mayonnaise-based salads and Jell-O. Yet toppings and dressings can be killers. "I don't see any vinegar and oil; the Italian dressing looks creamy...." So that meant I had permission to load up on the blue cheese. Was it my fault that the dressing poured out too quickly?

The best was last. The dessert was assorted cream pies: chocolate cream pie topped with whipped cream, lemon cream pie, and an Oreo cookie cream pie with a crust of Oreo cookies. The slices looked pretty thin, so I thought, "Maybe I should have a slice of each flavor." Sound familiar? I managed to choose a slice of Oreo cream pie and leave the buffet line. This is an example of "always eat dessert," but don't let your eyes be bigger than your stomach, as my mother would have said. In this case I knew I could polish off a slice of each pie. Good thing I was sitting with other people. I couldn't possibly eat three pieces of pie in front of somebody I didn't really know, or even worse, in front of a friend. Peer pressure was one reason I lost weight in the convent. I couldn't possibly eat a few slices of homemade bread and butter, I who was overweight, in front of the other girls. What would they think of me? "She's already fat and now she eats three pieces of bread with butter."

There is a lesson here. Even if you live alone, try not to eat every meal alone. The old "rule" we all recall is, "If no one sees you eat it, the calories don't count." That rule is, of course, wishful thinking. Gaining weight means living in a fairy-tale world of wishful thinking. This is why excellent diet programs, like Weight Watchers, encourage people to keep a record of what they eat. A lick of frosting here while icing the cake, a bite of meat there while cooking dinner to see if the meat is seasoned right....These things all add up. At Weight Watchers, people are encouraged to document what they eat for a while until they become more cognizant of all those extra bites slipped into the mouth.

Back to the buffet. I ate like this for about a week. Then it dawned on me as the rolls were forming over the waistband of my jeans that maybe I couldn't follow the Don't Be on a Diet in a Restaurant rule when I was going through the buffet line for three meals a day, seven days a week. I had to face the fact that I was eating at a buffet at "home" seven days a week, so I couldn't follow my holy habit of Don't Be on a Diet in a Restaurant. This had to be called "eating at home" for the two months I would be staying there. That's why I find it best to frequent a buffet-style restaurant almost never. I eat too much at buffets, so I cannot give advice. I just don't go.

For those people who eat out in a restaurant once in a blue moon, don't be on a diet while you're dining. For those of you who eat lunch out at work every day and dinner out as well one to three times a week, listen up. This is not about joining the convent, wearing a habit, and letting the mother superior dictate what you eat. This is about the habit of making good food choices when in a restaurant.

There are tiny habits I have developed through the years when eating in a restaurant that help save on calories so I can eat what I enjoy and not feel deprived.

BREAD

For starters, I don't have the discipline to tell the waiter not to bring the bread basket. *I try to space out my bread eating*: one piece as soon as the basket arrives at the table, because it looks so good I can't resist, and one piece with my salad. As the entrée usually comes with a starch, I generally don't eat bread with the meal. I try to make two pieces of bread my limit. I remember years ago being on a first date with someone, and when the bread basket arrived, I ate one piece of bread right after the other. My date commented, "Had I known you were going to eat an entire basket of bread before dinner, I could have saved money on your entrée by not ordering you one." (Ask me if I ever dated that guy again!)

If you are used to eating many pieces of bread with each meal, you will lose weight by eating only two pieces. If you are a small person, you may want to gradually cut back to one piece of bread. If bread isn't really your favorite thing, then skip the bread and save the calories for something else. Carbs are hard to pass up, so a little bit of bread could ward off a carb binge when you return home from the restaurant. If you can afford it, skip the bread and order a shrimp cocktail. If there is a choice, try to dive into the whole wheat rolls instead of the white bread rolls. Whole wheat bread is a healthier choice for most people *and* it's more filling!

Now, what about adding butter and/or olive oil to the bread? I love butter but was under the impression for years that olive oil was healthier and contained fewer calories than butter. Not true! We think of butter as a no-no loaded with fat, while we think of olive oil as a healthy food. Both contain things that are good for us. Olive oil also contains many calories, making it good for you but only in moderation. A tablespoon of butter contains 102 calories; a tablespoon of olive oil contains 119 calories. At a meal, we might use one pat of butter and think it's plenty; that's 51 calories. However, it's very easy to use two tablespoons of olive oil (238 calories) and think it's not enough. The difference: 187 less calories if you go with one pat of butter. That 187 calories is equivalent to what you get in four ounces of chicken breast meat—a whole entrée for the price of a little olive oil! Use the pat of butter on a 27- to 50-calorie slice of Italian bread and order a four-ounce grilled chicken breast as the entrée! That little savings of 187 calories every day represents 68,255 calories per year! On a common 2,400-calorie food allowance per day, choosing a pat of butter over two tablespoons of olive oil makes a difference of a month of meals in calories!

WATER

After the bread in a restaurant, I also start drinking the large glass of ice water just set in front of me. Water is your friend. That glass of water can be almost as filling as the bread. Try to drink at least one glass of water before or during the time you eat that first piece of bread. Drinking lots of water before and during your meal must become a habit at every meal. Growing up, we had water with every meal. My father, a medical doctor, always said, "Water is the best drink in the world." He never elaborated on *why* water was the best drink in the world, but we all drank a lot of it. One of my duties growing up was to fill a pitcher with ice water, fill everyone's glass with water while setting the table, refill the pitcher, and keep it on the serving counter next to my place at the table. (My mother and I both sat next to the serving counter.) During the meal, I refilled the water glasses of my father and brothers, and when the pitcher was empty, I went back to the sink to fill it again. We always had water on the table in the convent too. In this case, drinking a lot of water was a habit I brought *to* the convent and continued while there. Drinking water was my habit well before carrying a water bottle with us wherever we go became all the rage.

Only in later years did I wonder about the "why" my father never explained. Growing up, I guess I thought a lot like the little girl Kathy on the TV sitcom *Father Knows Best*, which I watched regularly. I identified with Kathy. In the case of drinking water, it was just a matter of "father knows best." Since then, I've learned a bit about why water is the best drink in the world. As this is a book about weight loss and maintenance, let's talk about why water helps us lose weight.

- Drinking a glass of water before diving into the meat and potatoes, whether at home or in a restaurant, is filling and makes us want to eat less. Our bodies are made up of about 60 percent water, according to the nutritionist guest speaker at the weekly marathon training classes I attended. We can go weeks without food but only days without water. So as we trained for our whole or half marathons, we all carried bottles of water as we walked. Make no mistake, I am no marathon runner, as noted previously. However, to date I have completed over 20 marathons—often I came in nearly last, but I finished!

- Water is something everyone can afford. It's important to me that everyone who wants to follow the Convent Diet as a lifestyle be able to afford my recommendations. The sisters take a vow of poverty. I follow in the sisters' footsteps with my dietary recommendations.

- Through my years of marathon training, I learned that water helps our muscles work better. Our postulant mistress knew what she was doing in more ways than one when she led us up and down the hills through the tangled briars and brambles on those muggy Midwest summer days. We came back to the convent looking for a glass of water!

- Water improves brain function. This is a rather intangible point. How do I know my brain is functioning better because I'm drinking water? Here is one little story that makes the connection between brain function and fluids very real. My mother spent the last two months of her life in a nursing home. She suffered from, among other things, normal pressure hydrocephalus, or water on the brain, a malady that can cause dementia. As Mother neared death and her body functions began to shut down, she stopped eating and, of course, stopped drinking. Her dementia seemed to become dramatically worse. Mother tried to hit me if I tried to give her water, help her sit up, and so forth. She became very agitated and called me "a little shit," a word I had never heard my mother use in her life. The nurses hooked Mother up to an IV filled with fluids. Within hours Mother was calm and I was no longer "a little shit." I then saw the stunning power of water.

- Drinking water can prevent and ease headaches. When I feel a headache coming on, I drink lots of water. Many times that will stave off the headache, and I won't need to take an aspirin. With the water, I'm getting rid of two things at once: a headache and extra pounds.

- I've been told that water is good for your skin and helps with all bodily functions. I drink a lot of water, so I don't know what my skin would look like without it. I leave the bodily functions discussion to the doctor.

- Drink water before a night of partying and martinis, and drink water before bed. Maybe that will ward off a hangover.

- Don't have a breath mint handy? Drink lots of water. A dry mouth can cause bad breath because there isn't enough saliva to rinse away the bacteria in the mouth. Prevent dry mouth and therefore prevent bad breath by drinking water.

In summary, drinking water can save a lot of money. I can't get that vow of poverty out of my head, it seems. You won't need to buy sports drinks for muscles, supplements for brain function, aspirin for headaches, laxatives for constipation, an expensive jar of skin cream for wrinkles, and mints and mouthwash for bad breath. Whether your water comes in bottles or from the tap is up to you.

Finally, there is scientific evidence that H_2O really does help you lose weight. Often cited is research by Michael Boschmann, MD, and colleagues at the Franz-Volhard Clinical Research Center in Berlin, that water consumption increases the rate at which people burn calories. The impact may be modest and the findings preliminary, but such research could have important implications for weight-control programs.

WINE

When the waiter arrives at my table, the next big decision is: Do I have a glass of wine, or do I stick to water? I love a glass of wine when I'm out for dinner in the evening, assuming I'm dining out only once or twice a week. If I'm out to relax and the evening is a little bit special, I order a glass of wine. If I'm dining out because I just finished the workday and there's no time to go home and cook dinner before I have to be at an evening meeting, I skip the wine for many reasons. The latter is not a dinner of relaxation; it is a dinner of convenience. I really notice right away a bit of weight gain if I've had two or three glasses of wine in a week, all else being the same.

First of all, a glass of wine is five or six ounces. This is about what is served in a restaurant as one glass of wine. However, most of us, when pouring a glass of wine at home, tend to be a little heavier-handed. At the convent, a glass of wine seemed to be something less than five ounces, and I never saw anyone pouring refills. And yes, wine is served in the convent for special occasions.

If your wine drinking is confined to a glass or two when dining out occasionally, drink your preference, white or red. However, there may actually be benefits to drinking red wine in moderation. A glass of red wine, I have read, raises the heart rate and metabolism, and therefore calories are burned more quickly. A good metabolism is helpful to weight loss and maintenance. Having your doctor check your metabolism could be a good idea. The body metabolizes alcohol before food, which means some of the food calories have the chance of turning to fat if most of the necessary calories are provided by those glasses of wine before the meal. While we're on the subject of calories, a glass of wine contains anywhere from 110 calories to 375 calories, depending on the size of the glass and the type of wine. Sweet wines have more calories than dry wines; simply, there is more sugar in sweet wines. However, dry wines contain more carbs. So pick your poison, so to speak. And finally, alcohol increases the appetite. That glass of wine before the meal may sabotage your best efforts to "be good" and eat the right type and amount of food during the meal. Remember that water, on the other hand, fills you up.

APPETIZERS

When you're at a restaurant, is it a good idea to order an appetizer? That depends. If that shrimp cocktail keeps you from eating the bread, then ordering an appetizer is a good idea. If the appetizer of deep-fried cheese balls is just a way of piling on more food and ordering more drinks, then forget about it. Salty food, like cheese balls, makes us crave more drinks. This is why many restaurants provide free appetizers during happy hour; it's really about selling more drinks, not largesse toward customers. If you order two appetizers such as shrimp cocktail and lettuce wraps to replace your entrée, then by all means go for the appetizers.

We did not have appetizers in the convent. The vow of poverty would preclude such frivolous spending. That thought is always in the back of my mind when I am at a restaurant. Skipping the appetizer if you are going to order an entrée is a good way to cut down on the size of the bill; eating two appetizers and no entrée may also be an economical way to go.

SALAD

Should you order salad or not? Sometimes I'm in a restaurant where everything is served à la carte and that salad is 10 dollars. If you can afford it, order the salad. It may be better to add to the bill than add to your waistline. If you don't fill up a bit on salad, it will be difficult to resist polishing off a 14-ounce rib-eye steak. (I am not writing here for the faint of heart. If you find the mere idea of eating 14 ounces of richly marbled steak in one sitting disgusting, then you may not need this advice.) Choose a salad you love so you will enjoy it. This is not punishment time. Or choose a salad jointly with your dining partner and share it.

If salad comes with your meal, eat it. If the entrée comes with a choice of salad or Boston clam chowder (the white, buttery, creamy kind), then here comes a dilemma. Let's say you really, really want the clam chowder but you know you *should* order the salad. What should you do? If you dine out rarely and the opportunity to enjoy the Boston clam chowder for which the restaurant is famous is a rare opportunity, order the Boston clam chowder. There may be other ways to compensate for that choice throughout the meal that won't really feel painful or like deprivation. Perhaps you're debating about whether to order the fillet of sole or the stuffed pork chop—go for the sole.

An average-size, simply prepared stuffed pork chop contains 500 calories, while a simply prepared, similar-size portion of fillet of sole contains 117 calories. This can make up the difference between Boston clam chowder and salad.

We must take a moment to talk about salad dressing. Do you normally ask for extra blue cheese dressing? A tablespoon of blue cheese dressing may have 210 calories, while that decadent cup of clam chowder has only about 230 calories. I like three tablespoons of blue cheese dressing on my salad; that's 630 calories—and we haven't even counted all that is in the salad! I'd be better off ordering the soup and saying, "Who cares?" Are you going to feel deprived having a salad with a tablespoon or two of low-fat blue cheese dressing, 20 calories per tablespoon? If the answer is yes, have the soup.

Another way to deal with salad dressing that may work for you is to ask the waiter to bring the dressing on the side. For example, at the convent, there were no oil-and-vinegar-based dressings, only creamy dressings. I love a thin Italian dressing. Full-fat is better, but I can handle low-fat, just not fat-free. Only the creamy kind of Italian dressing was available at the convent. I don't care for it. So I would take a small bowl and put a bit of blue cheese dressing in the bowl and dip my fork in the dressing before eating a bite of salad. There is nothing like the tossed salads served in fine restaurants, however. Another option is to ask for the dressing to be very lightly added. You'll probably eat more dressing this way, but such an approach may be a good compromise between lettuce drenched in blue cheese and a fork per bite dipped in blue cheese.

One more note on salad. Let's say you've eaten only half of your salad and the waiter brings the entrée. What do most of us do? We set the salad aside to be eaten with the meal or eaten later. What usually happens? We never finish that salad. Do we take the salad home in a doggie bag? No—which is okay. Soggy day-old salad is hard to eat. So, when your entrée arrives, have the waiter set the entrée to the side while you finish your salad. Eat all your salad and then take home some of that steak.

ENTRÉE

Entrée sizes have grown just as vanity dress sizes have shrunk. We are eating more and yet wearing smaller dress sizes. If you don't know that today's size eight is really yesterday's size 12, you may just keep eating. I wear dresses in a size eight. How is it that 40 years ago I weighed five pounds less than I do today and wore a dress size 12?

Back to entrées. If you are out for a special occasion or dine out only occasionally, choose the entrée your taste buds are craving. Even eat the whole thing—once in a while. If you're dying to bite into a juicy rib-eye steak but order grilled tilapia because you're on a diet, this will never work for a lifetime. If I'm really dying for steak, I order steak. If I order a 14-ounce rib eye and the normal recommended serving of meat is three ounces, I definitely try to take some home or split it with my husband. Splitting a meal is also easier on the budget than ordering two entrées. Having the entrée split in the kitchen before it is served to you will keep you from the temptation of eating the whole thing. Just remember, seven ounces of steak is still more than the recommended serving of meat. In the end, however, if you just can't bear the thought of sharing because you want to eat the whole thing, order the whole thing. Fill up on salad and veggies and you might be surprised to see that you will have some steak left to take home. Do not fall into the trap of thinking, "There are only four bites left; I might as well eat them. Four bites is too little to take home and too much to waste." Your waiter will not think you "cheap" for wanting to take home four bites of expensive steak. Besides, do you care what the waiter thinks? An even harder question: Do you care what your friends with whom you are dining think?

The good thing about going out to dinner with nuns is that I don't have to worry about any of these things. The nuns live with a vow of poverty and are on my side. Your friends? Maybe or maybe not. You don't want your friends to think: 1) You've become a little old lady asking for a doggie bag, 2) "Money must be tight; I would never take home four bites of steak, and if I did I would feed it to my dog," or 3) "If she's on a diet and doesn't want to finish her steak, why doesn't she just let the waiter throw it away? Is she obsessive-compulsive?"

It's hard to overcome this kind of self-talk, but do so. If you have friends who think any of these things, perhaps you don't need these people as friends. And you might actually be surprised to learn that your friend, who seems to have everything, applauds you for taking home those few bites of steak! While I recommend creating food habits and then not focusing on food, this is where it's good to be self-centered and focus on what's best for you. Take home that steak.

We all know that the size of restaurant entrées has increased over the years (see the graph). Many things have doubled in size. And many of us can eat the bigger-size restaurant entrées. We don't order just a hamburger at McDonald's; we order a Big Mac or a Quarter Pounder with Cheese. A McDonald's hamburger, like my grandmother used to order for us, has 250 calories. A Quarter Pounder with Cheese contains 563 calories, and that doesn't include a side of fries and a chocolate shake.

Entrée size at the convent 50 years ago was like the McDonald's hamburger of 50 years ago: small by today's standards. This is why portion control is so difficult in today's times. We are served so much food, and it is so easy to eat everything we are served. We don't need to enter a convent to find the correct portion of food, but we do need to look back at the portion size of 50 years ago and think about that as we dive into our order of spaghetti with meatballs. Or, as I said earlier, ask the waiter to box up half of your entrée before it is served to you.

How the entrée is cooked also makes a difference. Look for an item on the menu that is broiled or grilled. Broiled means that the entrée is cooked over a flame and the excess grease drips out below. If the menu says "grilled," ask how the entrée is grilled: over an open flame or on a grill plate? Over an open flame is essentially broiled. Grilled may mean that too, but it also may mean cooked on a grill plate. Like a sauté pan, a grill plate locks fat in, instead of the fat being cooked off. If grilled means on a grill plate, ask if you can have your meat broiled instead.

DESSERT

And now for the pièce de résistance. Generally, the word "diet" is synonymous with no dessert. But in the real world, most people could not live a lifetime with no dessert. And again, dessert doesn't have to mean a big slice of gooey, sticky pecan pie or a hunk of mud pie from the restaurant chain Claim Jumper. Now, if a restaurant you're at serves your favorite apple tarte tatin, which isn't available anywhere else in town, and you don't go to that restaurant very often, order the apple tarte tatin—or you will get home from dinner out feeling very deprived and you will probably raid the kitchen seeking any and every possible sweet in sight. This is a way to get off the path of good eating habits and onto the path of destruction.

If possible, select a light dessert, such as a scoop of ice cream (about 130 to 150 calories). Adding chocolate sauce will at least double the calorie count, so try not to add it. Berries make a good topping for ice cream, adding a lot of body and flavor without adding a lot of calories. Even if ice cream with berries isn't on the menu, it doesn't hurt to ask if some berries are floating around the kitchen. Better yet, ask for a bowl of berries topped with a large dollop of whipped cream. That whipped cream adds the feeling of decadence without adding a lot of calories. A cup of mixed berries topped with whipped cream may set you back only about 120 calories.

If none of the above works for you for dessert, and you really need to have a slice of apple pie (about 400 to 450 calories) or chocolate cake (350 to 450 calories for a twelfth of a cake), go for it. Again, remember that today's portions are probably double or triple what is considered a serving—a twelfth of a piece of layer cake, for example. Order that piece of cake in a to-go box and eat a few bites or half the slice and take the rest home with you; it's already in the box. How embarrassing would it be to order your cake in a to-go box and then eat the whole thing? Yes, this technique uses a bit of social pressure to help control portions.

After-dinner liqueur, anyone? On occasion, and a very special occasion at that, okay.

The last point in this restaurant discussion has nothing to do with food and everything to do with atmosphere. There is a great analogy between fine dining and convent dining that is worth mentioning. For most of us, enjoying our food in a leisurely manner is almost a lost art. There are many weight-maintenance benefits to both convent dining and fine dining in a restaurant. Here are some healthy dining tips from the convent. As you read them, think, "Fine dining in a restaurant." And then think, "I should bring these tips home with me too."

- Mealtimes were prescribed. There was no random rushing off to another activity. There were no 6 p.m. meetings or dancing lessons to attend. The end of the meal was signaled by the bell.

- The spiritual reading during the meal was soothing and worked well for digestion.

- The slow process meant reaching a satiated state after consuming less food.

- The atmosphere created by the lighting could be called dingy or it could be called soft lighting; take your pick. It wasn't like a sports bar with surround sound, TV lighting, and a cacophony, for sure.

- The main meal of the day was at noon, with a light supper served at about 6 p.m. No chance here for rolling into bed at midnight after an evening of three glasses of wine and half of a large pepperoni pizza.

- There were no seconds on most things most of the time—just the ever-present beckoning stack of homemade white bread.

Holy Habit #6

Opt Out of Diet Food: It Could Be Both Fattening and Expensive

I n the convent, as I've mentioned, we took a vow of poverty. We couldn't afford to eat organic lettuce and sugar-free ice cream. There were always commercial-sized cans of fruit preserved in syrup on the shelf and hot dogs in the large commercial refrigerators.

Not everyone can afford to buy special food. Not everyone has time to spend hours in the kitchen preparing string beans so they taste like pheasant under glass. The key is to eat what you like to eat, eat the foods that are familiar, and buy the food you can afford. Just make better choices within what you know. For example, I grew up in the Midwest eating lots of meat and potatoes. My parents also had a garden, so we had lots of beans, peas, and okra. If you grew up with similar food, instead of eating only the meat and potatoes and skipping the vegetables, why not try a couple of bites of beans and one less slice of meat and a smaller serving of mashed potatoes and gravy?

Here's a trick I learned that has been as crucial as Always Eat Dessert: Try the low-fat or nonfat version of whatever it is, maybe salad dressing or yogurt. If you can't tell the difference or don't mind the difference and the price of the item is in your budget—often the same as the full-fat version—then eat the nonfat or low-fat version. However, if the difference matters, then eat what you like. Here's my example: yogurt. I bought low-fat and nonfat yogurts and found that they just sat in the refrigerator because I didn't really like then. Then I tried Noosa full-fat yogurt because some samples of it were handed out after the Long Beach Half Marathon I had just walked. I loved it—the yogurt, not just the marathon. Now I buy Noosa full-fat yogurt and eat lots of yogurt. There are benefits to eating yogurt—full-fat or nonfat—for a lifestyle of healthy weight maintenance. Just be aware of the sugar added to flavored yogurts. I eat a lot of plain yogurt topped with fresh berries, seeds, and nuts.

The real question here is: What is diet food and what is not diet food?

What is not diet food: natural foods, mostly vegetables, such as carrots, celery, and radishes. Also what is not diet food: many prepackaged items, such as food prepared under the supervision of dietitians and offered to the public as part of a weight-loss program. There is nothing wrong with using a good crutch to help lose weight. Sometimes we need a jump-start; we need to see some quick results to encourage us to continue through the hard times of the weight-loss process. My personal weight-loss program of 50 years ago did not include a jump-start, because when I entered the convent I did not set out to lose weight. I was on what you might call an "accidental" weight-loss program. Upon reflection, I think that this has much to do with the reason I have kept my weight off all my life. The Convent Diet in many ways replicates this "accidental" approach to weight loss. The plan is positive, includes dessert, allows one to be a couch potato, and encourages focusing on more important things in life than food. However, "accidental" can never mean "an overnight miracle." I realize that most people set out on a deliberate journey to lose weight and want to see results quickly. Therefore, jump-start crutches as well as a few helping hands along the way can spell success. However, a crutch cannot be a lifestyle. Using a crutch can be a way to stay the course of your chosen lifestyle.

We commit to another person in marriage to stay joined for a lifetime. Sometimes we need the crutch of a vacation or a retreat to renew that relationship and stay the course. A teacher needs a sabbatical after a number of years, to step away, maybe write a book, refresh, and renew before returning to the classroom. The vacation and the sabbatical are crutches that help people stay the course. We do not perpetually live on vacation (no jokes here please). A sabbatical is not a life's career.

WHAT IS DIET FOOD?

There are processed foods out there advertised as diet or low-calorie foods that are simply empty calories. I'm not talking about the empty calories of sweets that provide little nutrients. As stated earlier, dessert is okay and for some people dessert may mean sugars.

Avoid fake foods such as diet cola beverages and anything containing artificial sweeteners. Do you love diet iced tea, sugar-free Jell-O, or sugar-free ice cream and cookies? Food of this nature shouldn't really be called food or even empty calories. These things are chemicals our body doesn't need, and they could even be harmful. Diet foods of this nature should not be a staple in your diet. Watch the labels: "fat-free" is not the same as "low-fat." Try to avoid processed fat-free foods; they may contain harmful chemicals. Low-fat is fine. Even be careful with yogurt, that special, healthy food many of us love and find good for us. Try to avoid the fat-free, low-carb yogurts. While they may help you slim down in the short term, they may also help make you sick or even kill you in the long term. There is no benefit to a slim corpse.

I am in no way a health food queen, but hopefully I learned some common sense in the convent and throughout the rest of my life. I am neither a doctor nor a registered dietitian, but those who are, are mostly against artificial ingredients).

I admit that as a former fat person, I have found that the fear of sickness and death from fake foods that are nothing but a pile of chemicals is often not enough to deter me from drinking a diet cola. Now my excuse for sticking to the diet version of cola is that I'm addicted to the taste and don't like the aftertaste of real cola. Of course, I shouldn't be drinking cola at all, but I do—just not very much. Again, depriving myself of things I like will only set me up for a lifetime of being fat. I *do* drink an occasional diet cola. Six lashes with a wet noodle for me. Every time I am tempted to say, "Do as I say and not as I do," I think of all the patients my father, a doctor, put on diets while he was himself considerably overweight. My father's saving grace was his sense of humor, so maybe that's what I am applying now to this topic. A sense of humor always helps. Don't take yourself too seriously.

However, the fact that new research is showing that these diet foods may actually cause us to gain weight gets my attention. Research on the connection between drinking diet cola and weight gain is limited and inconclusive. However, from my own experience, I can say that drinking a diet cola makes me feel like I have permission to add the cheese to my burger as well as a side of fries because, after all, I'm saving calories by drinking diet soda. That kind of thinking can for sure cause weight gain. Is the conclusion here that drinking diet soda causes weight gain? I don't think so.

I do know that buying these nonfat packaged diet foods adds a bundle to my already high grocery bills. At this point the cheapskate in me rears her ugly head. Saved by the vow of poverty!

Always Take Time for Yourself

"I don't have time to eat right and exercise" is a statement I hear all the time. I'm going to quote Sister Mary John Thomas again from freshman year in high school. When I told her I hadn't had time to do my homework, she said: "We always find the time to do the things we really want to do." Enough said.

In the convent, we were doing the things we wanted to do because we chose to be there. Just being there 24/7 meant we had found time for ourselves. Those who didn't want to be there simply went home. There were no bars on the doors and no recriminations. For the person leaving, it simply meant that taking time for oneself was a calling other than religious life.

The convent routine provided time for personal growth and education as well as for prayer, duties, and helping others. Occasionally nowadays, I go to the Holy Spirit Retreat house located about ten minutes from my office and take the course in "centering prayer." Keeping centered is about taking care of oneself. Taking care of oneself means finding time for the self. Taking care of oneself encompasses many things. Some of those things include keeping in shape, not just spiritually but mentally and physically. Finding time for oneself means finding time to "just be." Many people think the convent is only about prayer and penance and maybe even punishment. The convent is about becoming a whole person, becoming one with oneself, and enjoying the peace that brings to the self and so to all in the eyes of God. Only when we know who we are and are comfortable with ourselves can we help others and truly listen to others. A big reason for choosing religious life is the calling to help others. The only way a person can help others is to first be one with oneself. This is the global meaning of "take time for yourself."

Using this global meaning of "take time for yourself" tells us that in everything we do each day, we are taking time for ourselves. We are fully present in the moment. I'm always emotionally a happier camper at the end of a day filled with client- and people-helping moments than a day filled with paperwork, legalese, problems to solve, and technical issues. Being fully present in each moment is taking time for oneself in the global sense. Why do I feel so much more satisfied at the end of a day filled with client meetings than a day filled with paper problems and calling the plumber? Listening to those clients and being fully present with them is personally satisfying and therefore is its own kind of taking time for myself.

Former Harvard professor Richard Alpert, also known as the spiritual teacher Ram Dass, comments on this perspective of taking time for yourself. He states that "in the present moment, there is no time."

When I am at the convent nowadays, I work at my desk all morning. At noon, I go to one of the dining rooms for lunch. The food, as mentioned, is now served buffet style. There no longer are servers. With my tray filled, including dessert, I look out and head for a table with sisters whom I do not yet know. I think to myself, "What stories will I hear today? What mystery lies behind that face?" I am energized by the anticipation of hearing something new, of getting to know someone just a little bit—or maybe a lot. That will depend on the sister. I will go where the conversation takes me, interested in whatever is shared. Most often the "Where are you from?" and "What did you do?" questions lead to stories and reminiscing about the past, and often passions, points of view, values, thoughts of theology, and personal philosophies of life emerge. I leave the dining room and go back to work having been energized and enriched by the person who just shared herself with me. I consider that to be taking time for myself in the deepest way.

I never cease to be amazed by the energy and life in the words spoken by a sister who perhaps is bent over and can't see or hear very well. Inside that sister is youth, the relishing of today and the hopes and dreams for tomorrow. In some cases it's just the joy of being. I never think, "Oh, I've heard this story before," or, "What could I possibly have in common with her?" Each story is a gift to me of a bit of that person. I go back to work renewed by another's sharing. I am renewed because I was totally present in the moment. If time for oneself means a time for renewal, then I've taken time for myself by going to lunch and catching just a glimpse of the extraordinary mystery behind a smiling face of just one sister.

Regardless of whether a person is talking about things, people, or ideas, which Sister Marie told me are the three levels of conversation, all are about sharing a piece of the self. All are to be valued without judgment. I live in the moment preparing to receive whatever gift of self my table partner wants to share with me. All these types of gifts build friendship; thus we are in each other.

I take shared moments with new and old friends over lunch back to my desk and begin to write again, feeling renewed. What does taking time for yourself mean if not renewal? I am fully present in the now.

This is a starting place for busy people who have no time. Taking time for oneself in the traditional sense of spending an hour a day reading a novel or crocheting an afghan gives a traditional satisfaction. We feel disgruntled when we don't have that personal time. We feel put upon by others who interrupt us and take away our energy and self just a torn corner at a time. Being fully present in the moment suspends time and, if we allow it to, refreshes us.

Being fully present in the moment brings satisfaction and contentment. If we are content and satisfied, do we have an emotional need to overeat? Emotional eating implies frustration, unhappiness about something, anger, or even exuberance over an exciting event. Don't we go out to dinner to celebrate a birthday, a graduation, a promotion? Milestone events in our society often revolve around food. If we are calm and content, can't we enjoy the celebration over dinner without the second helping of each potluck item brought to the party? Stop and enjoy a dessert—just not five desserts.

The workday often brings stress. We go take a break from it all. What does that break include? A Snickers bar from the vending machine down the hall? Yes, there are times for snacks no matter how present in the moment, satisfied, and happy we may be. Enjoy the snack purposefully rather than accidentally. Be mindful of what you are eating. Are you really craving a Snickers bar specifically, or is that the snack choice that was "just there"? Be mindful and prepare: Bring in your purse or pocket a little baggie filled with an ounce of nuts, a cheese stick, trail mix—something you enjoy that will give you more energy than calories. If you have access to a refrigerator, bring some yogurt. Just a reminder that yogurt contains lactose, a milk sugar, which is easily used for energy. It also has a good amount of protein, which helps slow the absorption of that lactose, making the energy boost last longer.

I'm not going to say, "Take your break and go crochet for 20 minutes." When I take a break from work, I'm usually tired, so that break usually involves an energy-boosting snack. I prepare my snacks and bring them from home.

I never go to the vending machine. I always have "purposeful" snacks in my purse so that whenever I get hungry, wherever I am, I have something good to eat. And yes, sometimes I don't want anything I brought from home and I go to the vending machine and select the Snickers bar. But that is a mindful and purposeful decision and not a selection made by default because my purse was empty. If I know I'm going to spend the day at the mall or the evening at the theater, I have snacks in my purse. My husband counts on that too. During intermission at the theater, he will often ask what I've got in my purse. Being mindful, I try to carry items that my husband likes too, even if that means carrying chocolate kisses in the mix—but only one or two of them.

I remember studying the body's circadian rhythms in school. The term "circadian rhythms" refers to the body's internal clock and its movement. At what time of the day are you more energetic, and at what time are you in a slump? I slouch into a slump without fail about 3 or 4 p.m. each day. This is when I take a break and have a snack. I choose a snack that will give me energy both at the time and over the next few hours. Sugar gives an immediate high that does not last. Eat a candy bar at 4 p.m. and you'll feel energized, but by 5 p.m. the fatigue will return. Yogurt, for the reasons mentioned above, provides a more sustained boost in energy.

Understanding the science of snack choice and knowing how much renewed energy I need to do my job make for a more informed and mindful snack choice. I can usually pass on the candy bar because I know it won't help me feel the way I want to feel or *need* to feel to continue effectively with my day. Mindfulness here pays off most of the time.

Now let's talk about the kind of "take time for yourself" concept that is less global and more specific. This is the kind of "take time for yourself" we see articles written about in magazines because it's something we all crave but can't seem to do enough of; this is the practical "take time for yourself."

Someone says, "Mary, you're looking very tired and worn out. You need to take some time for yourself." What well-meaning friends are usually saying is, "Why don't you take time to go out to lunch with the girls, read a favorite Mary Higgins Clark mystery, or start tennis lessons?"

It's here that the subject of being an extrovert or an introvert walks onto the stage. We all appreciate quiet time, but the extrovert not so much. The extrovert recharges his or her batteries by being with others: going to a party, playing golf with friends, or going to a baseball game with the gang. The introvert, on the other hand, finds interacting with people exhausting. After a party, the introvert needs to return home to rest alone to recharge his or her batteries. The anticipation of going to a party may be overwhelming to an introvert, though he or she will enjoy the party while in attendance. As an introvert, I approach all group activities with a certain amount of dread, but I always enjoy myself when there. I'm always glad I went. But at a certain point, I want to go home and get away from the crowd. An introvert's renewal activities may include reading, listening to or playing music, and doing arts and crafts.

All people, whether introvert or extrovert, need personal time and their own space. My husband listens to me complain almost daily about having no time. Saying I have no time is my cry for the personal power to control my time and space. In reality, I have the power, but I need to perceive and believe that I have the power in order to be in control. A perception can be reality whether it is the objective truth or not. When I believe that my time is controlled by others, then it is and I feel stress. Yet my personal time is mine to control. My lack of ability to take control of my own personal time isn't about others, it's about me. I need to change my perceptions and the way I think about my time. Others will respect the message I put out there. All I must do is close my door, literally or figuratively, and take my space and time. If you present yourself to others as a doormat, they will walk on you, because you have invited them to do so. Instead of taking control of my own time and space, I just get so stressed that I feel like my head will explode. Then what? I eat, hungry or not, for comfort.

You need to empower yourself to find the courage to say, "After me you come first." (Quote stolen from my husband, who heard it often used in the financial services business and made it his own.) Ram Dass, in *Polishing the Mirror*, suggests that it may be easiest to find a few personal moments in the morning and again at night. For me this is true. By getting up a half hour earlier than necessary, I find a few moments to sit quietly before my busy day begins. Maybe I will read a few inspirational paragraphs, think about a meaningful quote, or write something. I struggle more to find that moment in the evening. I'm tired and my mind is filled with the chaos of the day. However, an after-dinner walk is my time to unwind. It is often a time of reflection and sometimes a time for a chapter of an audiobook on the subject of my choice. I have several audiobooks going at a time: motivational, meditative, how-to, and novels. I'm especially fond of murder mysteries. There's nothing like ending a busy day with a real cliff-hanger!

Taking that time during the workday is more difficult. What does it mean to do nothing, and does "nothing" always mean emptiness? To an onlooker, fellow worker, or boss, an observable posture of doing nothing may appear to be only wasted salary dollars. Seeing one in such a state often invites coworkers or the boss to intrude, thus making your time their time. Growing up, if I sat on the davenport seemingly doing nothing or reading a book, my mother saw this as an invitation to hand me a dust cloth and suggest that I make myself useful. "Make yourself useful" was one of Mother's favorite phrases. In the convent, such a posture of quietly doing nothing was considered meditation. I preferred the convent version of doing nothing. Meditation or thoughtful moments of doing nothing are probably best done on personal time.

Even a moment of solitude can provide a daily mini-vacation. By the time you are hanging by your teeth in despair, counting the days until vacation, it's already too late. Have you ever noticed that when you're in such a condition, a week's vacation isn't enough? You are so wound up, you need one week just to unwind before you even realize you are on vacation. You go back to work feeling as if you haven't had a vacation, while everyone at the office asks with a smile and anticipation, "How was your vacation?" Inside you seethe and think, "They don't understand."

It can be a challenge to let ourselves slow down. As Thomas Moore, author of *Care of the Soul*, says, "We seem to have a complex about busyness in our culture. Most of us do have time in our days that we could devote to simple relaxation, but we convince ourselves that we don't." It seems there is always something that needs doing, always someone who needs our attention. "Unfortunately," Moore says, "we don't get a lot of support in this culture for doing nothing. If we aren't accomplishing something, we feel that we're wasting time." Many of us learn the guilt of doing nothing early on in life.

Women in particular are often victims of the "I can't do nothing" syndrome. We are often programmed from birth to help others and put ourselves last. There is no end to the hours in the day needed to help others. There is then no self-time. Men are often programmed to be the breadwinner, to go off to work every morning, put in eight or ten hours, come home, and relax. Their job is finished for the day; with obligations met, personal time is now a man's birthright. These are two sexist generalizations, you say? For some yes and for many no. The convent dispelled this negativity about doing nothing and taught us the value of meditation. I visited with the nun who was the assistant postulant mistress in my day after many years of not having seen her, and I said, "Mary, what are you doing these days?" Sister Mary, long past official retirement age said, "I don't have to *do* anything. I just am."

I learned to find time for myself in the novitiate. Even there, we each brought our own backgrounds and biases. Were we receptive to what the novice mistress had to say? Maybe yes, because we were hungry for direction. Maybe no, because we were not ready to hear what was being said; we were teenagers who enjoyed getting away with breaking the rules. "Rules are for fools," as my friend Katy says. It was more fun to pull pranks than to listen. "Let's abduct one of the many statues of the Blessed Virgin Mary dotted around the convent and stick it on a fellow novice's commode and watch her howl in shock when she walks into the dorm, pulls back the curtain to her alcove, and sees the Blessed Virgin Mary looming large in front of her instead of her basin. Let's see if a professed sister will come running to check for disaster." Maybe the answer was no, because the novice mistress reminded us of our own mothers, seeming to have the very traits we disliked in our mothers. We were always on the wrong side of an argument with our mothers, so there was no way to be on the right side of the novice mistress's instruction. Maybe we were not receptive because the novice mistress had favorites, and they were not us. After all, most of us had just graduated from high school the month before entering the convent. Many of us were still kids. There will always be a world of favorites. As adults we say, "So what?"

This time of formation in the convent was a time for growing up, for getting the high school pranks out of our systems, for finding out who we were and how we fit into the convent life or if convent life was for us at all.

Whether we listened to or cared about the instructions we heard in the novitiate, we were given quiet time to ponder what we heard, to perform duties like buffing floors, cleaning toilets, or high dusting in silence, allowing our minds to focus on our instructions. At least that was the theory. Maybe it was just ineffective multitasking. Many of us did a lot of daydreaming instead of thinking or meditating. Those who stayed and took vows as well as those who left can attest to that! Did some of the stuff we heard in instructions stick anyway by osmosis? Perhaps. In my case, definitely yes. I was teased about having my head in the clouds and not knowing what was going on—as in, the latest pranks, who was the favorite, gossip, and all such typical teenage focuses. That was somewhat true. I lived in my own world of idealism and search for perfection. I made friends that have lasted a lifetime, but I was in no "group." I was neither the most popular nor the favored one, but it was only in hindsight that I learned the truth of that. At the time, I felt a general acceptance and lack of judgment about things like weight. I forgot that I was 50 pounds overweight. I had much more important things to think about.

We were trained to take time for ourselves so that we would then be filled with inspiration to share with others…to go out and conquer the world, as we would say today. Time for self doesn't mean finding an extra hour in the day and filling it with cleaning out the front hall closet, polishing the silver, or catching up on your emails.

Sister Marcia Allen, CSJ, (Congregation of the Sisters of St. Joseph) who recently gave a retreat at the convent, paraphrased the words of Thomas Keating, founding member and spiritual guide of Contemplative Outreach, in saying that there are three drives we all have during our formation as humans: 1) affirmation and affection, 2) safety and security, and 3) power and control. We go through a transformation of these desires in the quiet time of learning about ourselves. As true adults, we no longer need these things. We abandon them so we can give away these gifts. By giving these gifts to the unseeing and the undeserving, we claim our adulthood. In claiming our adulthood, we are able to let go of ego. We don't live in the past, because ego makes us captive to the past. The past allows us to let go; it empowers us to grow up and share.

This is the kind of "taking time for self" we experienced in the convent. By taking time for ourselves, we could learn to listen and help others, because we ourselves were now whole persons, grown-up sisters ready for vows, no longer young girls in formation energized by teenaged pranks.

This is why time for self is so important. It's growing time. It's time to become one with the self. Only if we are one with ourselves are we able to accomplish our most difficult, often unspoken, and most desirous goals.

Sometimes losing weight falls in this category of the unspeakable. We desperately desire to lose weight but cannot articulate it for fear of failure. We secretly order the weight-loss candies from Amazon or buy some sort of diuretic in the drugstore to give us a quick start on the task of losing weight. We don't tell anyone. We start in secret. If we fail, no one will be the wiser. While this is not a book on food addiction and while not everyone who is overweight is an addict, there's a little bit of that behavior in all of us who struggle with weight. Taking time for the self is invaluable for the relaxation of mind and body, for self-acceptance. Only in this frame of mind can we do what it takes, over the period of time it will take us, to lose weight. Only if we take time for ourselves for a lifetime can we keep the weight off for a lifetime. External weight-loss crutches can be good for the short term, such as subscribing to diet programs with prepared food, but we cannot eat that prepared food forever. At some point, we will go back to the foods we have always eaten. We need to find the strength inside of us to create the new habits necessary to go ahead and eat our usual and favorite foods but keep the weight off forever. Time for self helps us develop the strength to follow the first six of the Seven Holy Habits and really make them habits.

Daily Accountability Checker

W ant to make sure you are on track on a daily basis? Put this checklist where you can see it every day until it becomes a habit. There is one accountability check for each of the Seven Holy Habits:

- **Holy Habit #1—Visualization: You're Thin Until You're Thin.** Did I look in the mirror and visualize a "thin me" this morning? (Don't look as thin as possible? Wear something else today, but feel good about yourself before leaving the house.)

- **Holy Habit #2—Always Eat Dessert.** Did I keep my dessert size under control? (One serving of chocolate cake is not one-quarter of a cake.)

- **Holy Habit #3—Don't Count Calories, But Calories Count.** Did I skip that second serving of meat loaf by moving to dessert instead?

- **Holy Habit #4—Being a Couch Potato Is Okay.** Did I do something physical today in addition to chores and my usual daily routine? (Using a Fitbit or something similar might be helpful. Personally, I'm always looking to see if I got in my ten thousand steps each day, for example. If I'm a few steps short in the evening, I just walk in the bedroom while watching TV for a few minutes. It's a fun game to walk the ten thousand steps each day.)

- **Holy Habit #5—Don't Be on a Diet in a Restaurant.** Did I ask for a to-go box when I ate out at a restaurant...and did I put something in it? Secondarily, did I make good choices without sacrificing my desire for a favorite entrée?

- **Holy Habit #6—Opt Out of Diet Food.** Did I skip the unhealthy fake food, like the diet soda?

- **Holy Habit #7—Take Time for Yourself.** Did I take time out for myself today? I am number one in my book, and I can't help anybody else unless I take care of myself first. (Remember, even the airlines say that in an emergency, put your own oxygen mask on first and then help your child.)

PART IV

UPON REFLECTION...
WHAT I HAVE LEARNED

Where It All Began

oday is the start of my sixth day here at Mount Carmel for the second time, where "it" all started. "It" was not only the beginning of the 50-pound weight loss that changed my life but also the formation, as the daily instructions of young novices was called, of Mary Lou Reid as the person I still am today, 52 years later. As I walk these corridors again, corridors greatly changed, remodeled, and adapted to the needs of primarily older sisters now, I feel so grateful for everything given to me by the sisters.

My husband suggested I come back here to finish my book, as I was complaining about no time and constant interruptions, all great excuses for not writing a book. I was so excited when the plane landed and Sister Mira, whom I consider to be one of my best friends, picked me up and took me to dinner at an elegant Thai restaurant. I indulged in curry, rice, and wine, all major favorites. I of course practiced Holy Habit #5, Don't Be on a Diet in a Restaurant. My arrival was the night before Holy Thursday, so all I did for the first four days at the convent was eat, party, and pray, probably in that order. If I'm not careful, my excuses for not writing here will include two-hour meals visiting with old and new friends, a host of education classes from painting to history, and long walks exploring the grounds, enjoying the spring flowers. We don't really have four distinct seasons in Southern California, where I live, so I am relishing this change of season from the brown twigs of winter to the green buds of spring.

That first dinner on Holy Thursday was not just about beef tenderloin, beer-battered shrimp, sautéed baby asparagus spears, red roasted smashed potatoes, salad, and pomegranate cheesecake (all good reasons not to be on a diet); it was about sitting down at a round table filled with 50-year friends and acquaintances and window views of Iowa's rolling hills. It seemed we "girls" (all now 69 or older) couldn't talk fast enough.

The four days of Easter liturgy engaged me on a level I may have forgotten these past few decades. As a music major, I appreciated the angelic singing of the schola, all women in their seventies, eighties, and nineties. Closing my eyes convinced me that I was listening to young women in their twenties and thirties....How could that be? Are there a purity and simplicity of soul that express themselves in song? The use of organ, piano, guitar, and trumpet artfully woven throughout the words of liturgy encouraged me to take a deep breath, relax, join in the singing with my lately never-used cracking voice, and pray. My arrival at Mount Carmel was perfectly timed to prepare me, soul and body, to write. Much of the 24/7 work fatigue is falling away today, two days after Easter. I'm adjusting to the time-zone change and breathing deeply again. My eyes are seeing the simple joys of nature and the lives of the sisters around me. My daily business problems seem far away. Thank God my email is down; I don't have to feel guilty about not checking it!

Last night Sister Mary Jean invited me to join a little group that meets after dinner in one of the turrets (round-shaped rooms lend themselves to meetings and communication) for "centering prayer." Periodically throughout my financial planning career I would take time out for a centering prayer class at The Holy Spirit Retreat Center, just to get back on track. The group here meets at 6:25 p.m. "We don't say anything," said Sister Mary Jean. At 6:25 one of the sisters sounded a small gong, gave a brief invocation, and then there was absolute silence for about 20 minutes, with the gong ringing again to indicate the end of the session. I wondered out loud why the group was so small, and Sister Mary Jean said that many of the members had died. The group lost its leader to death last week. Could that be why no one said anything? The leader had been lost?

My personal 20 minutes of centering prayer consisted of simply trying to empty my head of things stressful and unnecessary. Is that prayer? Meditation? Does it matter? I can only start from where I am and move along the line of improvement. This is all we can do about anything: Start from where we are and move forward, not worrying about the steps backward that will invariably occur. This premise holds true with the process of losing weight and maintaining weight loss, the subject of the book I am here to finish writing. To maintain weight loss for a lifetime, what we do must become and remain a habit. The only way to develop a habit is to start from the beginning, which is wherever we are today. If you are used to scooping up large first and then second helpings of everything at meals and snacking in between meals, you cannot expect to immediately downsize to three peas on a plate and no snacks, so to speak.

BEING CENTERED AND BALANCED

I woke up this morning, remembered where I was (in a guest room in the convent), and got up looking forward to my day. I opened the drapes and just stared out for a few minutes. A red cardinal was sitting on a bare tree branch in front of my window. I had seen a cardinal yesterday in the same tree and marveled at the bright red color. I don't see cardinals where I live in Southern California. Swarms of large black birds with wide wingspans are circling overhead and landing atop the peaks and cross of the motherhouse directly outside my window. Are they crows? It's overcast today, in sharp contrast to the bright sun of the past few days.

I am reminded of Genesis 1:3: "Then God said, 'Let there be light,' and there was light." A cloudy day to me is still a day of light. Every day spent in a peaceful and welcoming place is a day spent in light. Light enables you to see more clearly your purpose and direction. Away from the darkness and chaos of a demanding schedule, my mind opens to allow creativity and focus to filter in like rays of sunlight. Is this my time of centering prayer? Being centered is not about religion. It's about coming to a place of interior silence. It's about openness. I'm neither a theologian nor a philosopher. I can only say what "staying centered" means to me.

I have lived among peoples of many different cultures and religions in my life. While I grew up in the Midwest, I have spent most of my adult life in either New York or Los Angeles. I have never lived in the South. Those I've come to know through the years with or without words share my longing to be centered. Creating space within brings openness to others and different ways of thinking. When I was still in school, my family took in a foreign exchange student from Turkey. It was amazing to me that Orhan could speak fluent English, which was his third language, after Turkish and German. What a different way of seeing the world and dealing with people and values Orhan had compared to my own. Orhan thought it only right and of course humane that if someone stole something, his or her hand should be cut off as punishment. I thought that to be horrifying at the time. As I got to know Orhan, I saw him as a very centered person within his own culture and value system.

Does being centered mean being well-balanced, or is the idea of being well-balanced simply a myth? Do you calculate balance on a daily, monthly, yearly, or lifetime basis? On a daily basis, being well-balanced is fiction. While it's important to set a daily schedule, following that schedule may also be fiction if you live out in the world with other people and have a career, a family.

My goal has been to write every morning for an hour. Some days I just cannot get up early enough to accomplish that goal. The phone rang at 7:30 one morning; it was an insurance company representative calling from New York at 10:30 a.m. who forgot that in California it was only 7:30 a.m. Another time I was in deep thought, doing research, and the phone call was from the daughter of a client letting me know her father passed away. On a lifetime basis, a balanced life being a centered person is essential. Yet days of interruption have a way of evolving into weeks, months, and years of interruptions unless you are proactive about being centered. As I learned in the novitiate during formation, I have to get my act together (not exactly the words used by the novice mistress) to be prepared to go out into the world and help others. I have to know myself and help myself first.

As I have said before, what are we told on an airplane in case of an emergency? Put your own oxygen mask on first and then help your child. To accomplish a goal, you must be in the season of life in which that goal takes a front seat.

The sisters have the right idea in using retreats to restore and rejuvenate themselves so that they may go back and better serve those with whom they work. As I described earlier, I've walked marathons and half marathons periodically over the past 15 years to raise money for charitable organizations. Those long walks help me restore and rejuvenate myself. I enjoy observing the seasons change as I walk weekly through Griffith Park. Walking is a centering time for me. I come back home to my husband a better, more relaxed wife. I finish the walk feeling renewed as a person with more energy to help others, with more creative juices flowing. Exercise is merely a by-product of doing something enjoyable that gets me moving, but a welcome by-product. Although my life is not about exercise and weight loss, I accomplish both by doing something physical that I enjoy. You've already read more about this in the section on Holy Habit #4, Being a Couch Potato Is Okay.

Being centered and balanced is the key to losing weight and keeping it off. Lifetime weight loss has to be a lifestyle, not a diet. That gets us to Holy Habit #6, Opt Out of Diet Food. That ties in with the phrase, "I'm going on a diet," which assumes that the speaker will also "go off the diet" at some point. Going off the diet is for most people the beginning of gaining the weight back—and more. Permanent weight loss requires a lifestyle change and then a permanent addiction to the new lifestyle. That's why maintaining weight loss has to be done by developing positive habits. No one can live a life of negativity and deprivation, which is many people's description of "diet," and many people think of what we eat to lose weight as "diet food." Instead, I look forward to eating that piece of apple pie after dinner, which gives me the strength not to take seconds on meat and potatoes. It was easier in the convent not to take seconds because there were no seconds. You don't have to enter a convent to develop the habit of eating seconds sparingly. I've been out of the convent for 45 years and usually do not eat seconds (unless the entrée is two peas on a white plate, so to speak). There are many who say that sugar is bad for us; probably true, but if a little bit of sugar is what it takes to help you eat less food, then such a crutch is okay.

Weight maintenance is not an all-or-nothing proposition. Maybe I ate too many cookies because *they were there for the taking*; they were just out of the oven and they were my favorite—peanut butter. So what? Tomorrow is a new day. When those cookies show up for lunch again tomorrow, they won't be so warm and fragrant. You will already have filled up on them the day before, and you know they will be available every day, so now it's easier to eat one cookie less. Gradually, instead of eating a dozen cookies after lunch, you will be satisfied with two cookies because you developed the habit of always eating dessert. No one can go from eating a dozen cookies after lunch to eating no cookies after lunch and maintain that for a lifetime. If two cookies is what you normally eat and you want to lose weight, develop the habit of eating one cookie. Over time you will lose weight. You will know that one cookie is your limit.

Of course, there are cookies (small vanilla wafers), and there are cookies (almost-Frisbee-size chocolate chip disks). While I don't recommend counting calories, something also almost impossible to do for a lifetime, calories do count. (You've read more about this in the section on Holy Habit #3, Don't Count Calories, But Calories Count.) Think "average-size" cookie. An average chocolate chip cookie might be three inches in diameter and have 300 calories. For comparison, an average slice of apple pie (an eighth of a pie) has about 300 calories. Eating even a few less calories every day will result in weight loss. One less cookie after lunch may be all it takes to maintain rather than gain weight.

I can't stress enough the importance of creating habits for yourself. Your habit may be: Always eat one cookie for lunch. Two cookies isn't bad, but you want to save room for dessert after dinner as well as after lunch. I'd rather have one cookie for lunch and then a piece of pie at dinner. This is the "stretch things out" trick. I do this all the time. I take some of my restaurant lunch to-go and have the leftover portion for dinner. Restaurant portions are huge, but believe me, I can eat them! Not a great habit to get into. Have you noticed that you seem able to eat more and more food at one sitting? That can come from eating too much restaurant food, too many seconds, too many buffets, or even too many cookies. Please see Holy Habit #5, Don't Be on a Diet in a Restaurant, for more on this topic.

FINDING MOTIVATION

This morning I'm reflecting on both the power and the emptiness of words, in the context of Holy Habit #7, Take Time for Yourself. My morning reading today didn't really speak to me, yet two paragraphs I read yesterday energized my entire day. I'm sitting quietly and I see the cardinal in the budding tree in front of my window again. The sky is gray and there are raindrops on my window, probably from an overnight shower. I read three more suggested scriptures for today; I still feel uninspired.

How many times do we get up in the morning and think only of getting ready for work, of getting the kids ready for school, and jump into the day's hustle and bustle with no reflection? The actions are all done from habit. But at some point, those actions required thought because they were not habits. Change requires thought and deliberate action until the habit sets in. The same is true when we decide to lose weight and in the same breath vow that "this time I will keep the weight off forever." We have spoken words to ourselves. In the beginning, they are merely words. Putting the words into action takes energy and motivation. Perhaps after saying these words to ourselves, the next step is to say the words out loud. Tell your spouse, your children, your friends, and everyone with whom you engage in conversation: "I'm going to lose weight, and this time I'm going to keep the weight off forever." Speaking these words out loud is an action step. There are so many sayings related to this process: "Put your money where your mouth is"; "She is a woman of her word"; "She's a real doer"; "She's all talk"…

Once we say it out loud, our words develop a life of their own. We have just created accountability. We are now responsible in the face of the world, at least to the people in our world, for losing weight and keeping it off forever. It's not good enough to say, "I'm going to lose weight; I'm going on a diet." Without adding the second part of the sentence "...and keep it off forever" we have made only half of a promise to ourselves and to our loved ones.

It often helps to examine the motivation behind the words. I see two women out for a walk together on the path below my window in this moment. What is their motivation: good health, weight loss, friendship bonding time, all three, or something else? I cannot presume to know the answer. We often assign motivations to others for their actions, and we are often not correct at all. Fear of what others think can keep us from taking a desired action. Motivation is very personal, and there are no right or wrong answers. I may say to someone, "The doctor says I should lose weight, so I'm going on a diet." This is usually not a strong motivation because it's coming from the outside, not from within. You may tell your friends that you're going to lose weight because you are getting older and may develop some health problems because of the weight—all very acceptable. Maybe deep down you are worried that your spouse is losing interest in you, a motivation not to be spoken out loud.

There are usually multiple motivations for the actions we take. Positive motivations are stronger than negative motivations. How about, "I want to lose weight out of love for myself" as opposed to "because my spouse might not love me as much anymore"? Only when we truly love ourselves can we love others and in turn become truly lovable to others. This is a lesson I learned over 50 years ago during our formation period as young sisters. Sometimes I forget that lesson and need to stop and center myself again, to take time for myself, Holy Habit #7. Self-love is necessary to being a whole person, and it is only in this state that we can help and love others. "I want to lose weight and keep it off because I love myself."

From there you may layer on other motivations: "I want to be healthy and have more energy, I want to fit into my favorite fashions, I want the admiration of family and friends, I want my husband to feel proud of me when he introduces me to his business associates," and many more. The outside world may cry vanity, old-school antifeminist, self-involved, or "That's great!" None of it matters because you love yourself, know who you are, and are comfortable in your own skin. Some things you can keep to yourself, and some things you may share without worrying about what others think, because you are in the driver's seat. You love yourself and are in control.

Shout from the mountaintops: "I'm going to lose weight and keep it off forever!" You will be amazed at the support structure and fan club that develop around you. I believe that by nature most people want to do the right thing; most people want to be helpful. I am here writing from the convent. I sit with the sisters for lunch and am universally wished well in my writing. I'm also peppered with questions: "What are you writing about? How it is coming along? Do you need anything to help you?" As you walk down the road toward perpetual weight loss, those close to you will want to help, will want to be kept in the loop regarding your progress and will empathize with your setbacks. Yes, there will be setbacks. If you truly love yourself, you will have the strength to overcome the setbacks and continue down your path toward success. Those around you will empathize and urge you on toward your goal. If you encounter people who seem to relish your setback, saying things like, "It's okay, we love you the way you are; you don't have to lose weight," or, "I gave up myself on trying to lose weight, so it's okay," find new friends. Of course, people who love you, love you the way you are now, but at the same time, they should support and encourage you to become the new you that you want to be, because that is your goal.

There is a theory of weight loss floating around today that "God wants you to be thin, so you must be thin to be loved by God." Nonsense. I believe in a loving God who loves us whether we are fat or thin. Such an external and concocted motivation to lose weight cannot work for a lifetime. So too, the passive-aggressive feigned support of "friends" in a lack of weight loss will not deter us if we truly love ourselves and if the motivation to lose weight and keep it off forever comes from within.

CHANGING WITH THE TIMES

This morning I squint as I look out the window; the rising sun is so bright. As I close the drapes partway, I see all the changes in the vegetation, the new building, and a new house on the grounds. So many years of a money shortage in the community meant selling off a bit of the land to support the sisters, and now there is a family or two seemingly living on "our" grounds.

As Bob Dylan wrote and sang, the times they are a-changin'. That Dylan song of the same name was a big hit in 1964. I played it on my guitar and sang it in high school, and as a young novice did the same in the convent. The war in Vietnam was raging, college campuses were filled with protestors, the hippies decorated the streets of San Francisco with psychedelic art, and the Church was reeling from the changes brought by Vatican II.

Is today much different? College campuses are certainly filled with pro-testors. California is still in turmoil—I know; I live there. And the Church is airing out its closets after pedophile scandals.

Am I the same girl I was when I was singing the Dylan song, or am I somebody different? The answer is, I am both the same and different. Sitting at the dinner table my first night here, I was with "girls" from my set. I asked myself: Who are all these old ladies sitting at my table? In my mind's eye, we're a gaggle of girls enjoying each other's company, and in reality, we are 70-year-old women, give or take, with many accomplished roles: treasurer of the community, secretary, vice president, president, and me, a Certified Financial Planner of many years. We are who we've become: women with the same core values, with many accomplishments to list on a résumé. It's the sameness that helps us bond and the diversity among us that stimulates and challenges us. I am welcome here even though I haven't been a sister for many years. These sisters live in a community that welcomes the world, same and different. We share the same God. The community practices hospitality, welcoming all who need to stay.

I walk from one building to another without going outside. The build-ings are now all connected to each other, with a new building between the old allowing for this connection. "New" means built in the 1980s, as compared with the original motherhouse in which I lived, studied, and worked so many years ago, built in 1892. The motherhouse is no longer filled with hundreds of young postulants and novices. It is currently a home for retired sisters. The new building provides assisted living, and the infirmary, as we called it 50 years ago, is now a nursing home for sisters. The generalate, where the mother general and the officers of the community lived and worked, has undergone a name change and, while it still provides office space, also provides hospitality for guests. There are newly built townhouses on the grounds, in the circle, as they say, for sisters who are still working. The buildings are like the people who inhabit them. They are filled with women of many ages, but the young-est, like the newest building, are no longer really young.

I marvel at how each building has changed while still keeping its origi-nal character. The second floor of the motherhouse—which used to be the dorms, each large room sectioned off by curtains, creating individual spaces large enough for a twin bed, a simple four-drawer dresser, and enough space for one person to dress, called an alcove—no longer exists as dorms. Each floor has been converted to individual bedrooms. An old space has been repurposed and modernized, keeping the integrity of the building intact.

Can't we describe a well-centered person the same way? We change with the times and grow from within, but the integrity of who we are remains intact. Though we are all older now, like these buildings we inhabit, the renewal process inside never stops. Change is difficult, but it must be embraced because the alternative, living in the past, is not an option. The past is gone, and all efforts to live there are only foolish. The sisters here are not living relics; they are engaged human beings centered by core values and a love of God and tolerance of diversity. The daily experience of walking here among these sisters centers me in the moment while giving me the energy, hope, and fortitude to work toward the future. I live in the today while envisioning the tomorrow and smiling at all that the past has fashioned inside of me.

LEARNING FROM THE PAST

It's a beautiful sunny day today, with temperatures in the low 70s. I opened the window in my room for the fresh air and to hear the singing of all the birds outside. There's a bird's nest in the tree in front of my window.

Since it's Sunday, I decided to take a long walk around the grounds. I took a few pictures along the way, looked at buildings and sites, and thought about the past as well as this moment. How important is it, I wonder, to hang on to the past? If you asked my mother that question, she would say in a heartbeat, "Forget about it." I don't think that is the correct answer. I think it's important to bring into the present those things from the past that make a difference in our lives. How lucky I am to be able to return to the same convent structure I entered 50 years ago. There is stability in that. But is the convent the same as it was in 1965? Not really. On the outside, other buildings now adjoin the 1890s motherhouse. On the inside much has been repurposed, modernized, and expanded. In a way, this is all perfect; it's the same but totally different.

We can say that many things in our lives are totally the same but different. My friends of 50 years are the same because they are still my friends. Yet we have all grown and aged, and our friendships have evolved. We really live in the moment knowing that the moment contains all that was good about the past. The brain has a wonderful way of being able to forget a lot of what was bad or painful in the past.

This connection we have with the past is essential in developing good habits. It takes time to develop a habit, so how grateful we can be for memory. Habits can be both good and bad. The good ones are difficult to develop, and the bad ones are difficult to discard. This is why it can be so difficult to develop the Seven Holy Habits for permanent weight loss initially. While you are developing the good habits, you may be fighting to discard the bad eating habits. Do you love to sit after dinner with a bag of potato chips and dip, as I did while I did my homework? Maybe you enjoy nibbling on these salty disasters while watching television or working on the computer or reading a book.

Some people can cut out a bad habit cold turkey, as they say. If that's you, go for it. Maybe the rest of us just need to eliminate potato chips and dip from the house. Young children don't need to develop potato-chip-and-dip-type eating habits. Remember, you are not on a diet. You are embarking on a new way of life, and your family will be grateful in the long run to join you on that journey. For adults living in the house, let them make their own snack choices with their own money. Make sure they don't share their chip-and-dip snacks with you! While we can guide our children, we cannot control the choices of grown children and other adult family members with whom we live.

In the convent, what we ate was controlled for us—to a point. Where there's a will there's a way, as the saying goes. I've heard stories of sisters sneaking down to the kitchen for ice cream. The supply of homemade bread was practically limitless. There were sisters in my group who gained weight in spite of the food controls. Are you going to sneak down for ice cream while you are working to develop the Seven Holy Habits?

MONUMENTAL MOMENTS

For the past two days, I've been the only one on my floor here at the convent. Two new sisters will be here tonight, however. Once I realized I was alone on the floor, I knew I could leave my dishes as they were in the kitchenette while I went to a centering prayer session, and no one would notice or be inconvenienced by my mess. I had my choice of TV channels in either the lounge room or the kitchen. I could play music in my room as loudly as I liked, knowing I wouldn't disturb anyone. I could eat ten cookies if I wanted to, and no one would see me do it. I could eat *anything* I wanted to, in fact, and no one else would see me. Remember the phantom rule that says, "If no one sees me eat it, the calories don't count?" We all wish…

This is the circumstance for losing weight and creating a lifestyle of keeping it off that those who live alone have. I lived alone for many years, and yes, was able to hone and practice my Convent Diet lifestyle of eating just the right amount to maintain a steady weight without interruption.

However, ten years ago I married and things changed. I cooked lots of pasta for my Italian husband, which, of course, I ate myself. We went out to dinner all the time in celebration of our new life together. We sat around in the evening watching TV together on the davenport. Both my husband and I "suddenly" gained weight. I married late in life, and my husband is three years older than I am, so we weren't young. (A discussion of weight and aging deserves its own chapter and probably its own book.) It was all great fun but suddenly we both realized that we needed to settle into a new lifestyle together, one that would work for the long term.

There are monumental moments in all our lives, such as marriage, a new baby, going back to school, a new job, and retirement. Each monumental moment involves change. A good habit must weather change, must be practiced through the change. A bump in the road must be hopped over; we must carry on. The Seven Holy Habits for permanent weight loss and weight-loss maintenance must be just that: habits. Accept the bumps in the road, appreciate the monumental moments, but keep the weight-maintenance habits running like beautiful music in the background.

CREATING COMMUNITY THROUGH MEALS

During Passover this year, one of my favorite clients and friends, Bill, passed away. For me as a Christian, Bill's actual day of death was Good Friday. His last night with us was Holy Thursday, a night during which Christians around the world commemorate the last Passover meal Jesus shared with his friends. So began a Christian tradition that was already a sacred ancient Jewish tradition. The sharing of this tradition expresses my bond with my Jewish friend, Bill, as well as the bond of many traditions that Christians and Jews share around the world. We gather and share a meal; we create community. The meal feeds not only our hunger for food but also our hunger for friendship and bonding with others. I like to think of Bill as having been there not only for his Passover but for my Holy Thursday, sharing what was for Bill a last meal. Bill will always hold a place in my heart even as the sadness of his death passes with time.

If a family is too small for a whole lamb, it shall join the nearest household in procuring one and shall share in the lamb in proportion to the number of persons who partake of it. (Exodus 12:4)

ADJUSTING

Miss Italy and Miss Poland, aka Sister Therese and Sister Joan, have just moved to third-floor Marian Hall, from assisted living to nursing care. They are inseparable friends who look out for each other. Together they appear to be the female Laurel and Hardy, and they're just as funny.

Sister Therese has 20 percent kidney function, and Sister Joan's diabetes is out of control.

Sister Joan has been receiving a shot for 30 years, but every day forgets her shot—she's always off somewhere escaping the nurse. When they can't find her, they always think Sister Therese should know where she is, but sometimes no one can find either of them. Sister Joan's blood sugar level runs up to 400 without her shot.

Sister Therese is overweight. She has always lived the life of a good Italian: lots of pasta. Over lunch she tells me that she lost 20 pounds at Weight Watchers but gained ten back in six months.

That's better than saying she should go to the gym in the Wellness Center and never doing it. Neither Sister Therese nor Sister Joan can get used to the more controlled environment at Marian Hall, with its skilled care. They smile about it, pay lip service to the necessity of it, but practice their Houdini disappearing act when they can. How are these two adjusting to skilled care? They're trying.

CHANGING LANDSCAPES

I woke up this morning, opened the drapes and saw—could it be?—snow. This is April 27. I wondered if it could be blossoms falling from a large tree nearby, as daily the blossoms have been turning into green leaves and daily I have enjoyed this wonder of nature, something I do not see in arid, seasonless

Southern California. The snow isn't sticking; it lands and seemingly evaporates. I check the weather forecast on my phone and learn that it's currently 37 degrees and raining. Ah-ha…this is *rain*. I immediately worry about the tulips, the daffodils, the lilacs, and so on. Will they be ruined?

The birds come and go as usual from the tree in front of my window. I look for my friend the cardinal, who has kept me company almost daily. I see a robin land on the very top branch. Another robin joins it. What a delight it is to watch birds I don't see in my backyard in Southern California. I also see crows with their broad wingspans flying above. We have lots of crows in my backyard…so many that we also have a large plaster owl hanging over the patio.

This is the first really cold and rainy day I've experienced in the two weeks I've been here. I was just beginning to think that the wool sweater and turtleneck I brought with me were a waste of suitcase space. I turn up the heat in my room and put on some socks because my ankles are cold. Somehow it all feels so cozy. I sit high up in front of a big picture window in my bathrobe sipping hot coffee, enjoying my beautiful, ever-changing view. As my desk faces the window, on a rainy day like this, I can work on my computer without glare and without having to draw the drapes closed. I cherish these early mornings. My mind is open and fresh. It's too early for the phone calls from California, bringing work issues with them, to start coming in.

How blessed I am to be here in the convent among friendly and welcoming sisters. I wonder briefly why I ever left the convent. I know that if things then were as they are today, I might not have left. Like everything, convent life has evolved and changed over the past 50 years. Just as the newer convent buildings contain more outlets for hair dryers, something not needed when we wore the habit, convent lifestyle has relaxed and become modernized. Friendships are encouraged and nurtured, and the uniform that was the habit is gone. The lifestyle here is not so uniform either. The phrase "behind the convent walls" now has no meaning. This convent is no longer exclusively a teaching order; all professions, including teaching of course, are represented by the sisters today. There is a sister who had been the mayor of Dubuque. There are sisters doing mission work in South America; there are sisters who are attorneys fighting for social justice, and much more. Had I entered just a few years later, might I have been a sister with a financial planning practice, as I have had for the past 30 years? Yet my relationship with the many sisters who are dear friends has been a constant thread running through the 50 years since I entered the convent. In many ways, I have never left the convent. The influence of the sisters and this lifestyle has molded my life.

Yet I immediately remember my loving husband and all that fills my life back home. How many people have ever had the opportunity to live in two such worlds at once?

RECOGNITION LEADS TO CHANGE

Change is the only constant in life. Every morning I draw open my drapes wondering what the change in the weather will be that day. In fact, today appears to be a repeat of yesterday...and the day before...and the day before: cloudy, rainy, and windy. At first, I wish for warmth and sunshine. Then I accept the weather and continue with my day, putting the weather in the background.

This morning I pass a woman in the hallway on the way to the shower, greet her with a smiling "good morning," as I would any stranger, walk a few steps, and turn around. In fact, we both turn around at once and say each other's names. We haven't seen each other in many years. We have both changed with age to the point of a lack of recognition in the first moment. Then we see the person we have each always known. The changes don't matter; we are still who we are behind the physical changes.

I upgraded the Office suite on my computer two days ago from Office 13 to Office 16. I'm fighting the change, because it no longer has the comfort of familiarity. I have to learn a few new things in order to use the program, and I can't write without the program—at least I don't want to write without the program. If thrown on a desert island, I could always write in the sand, but let's not go there.

Here are three examples of change that have crossed my path in moments: 1) the weather, 2) an old friend, and 3) technology.

In the first instance, I long for change. I'm tired of the gloomy weather. Every morning I wake up excited by the prospect of changing weather: spring blossoms turning to leaves, trees no longer looking like sticks, now so full of leaves I can't see the pine walk through the trees in front of my window anymore. I take the weather as it comes. There are little joys to be found in each type of weather presented to me. I not only accept the changes; I relish them. And after a few moments each morning I put thoughts of the weather on the back burner and begin to tackle the important things in my day.

The same is true with maintaining weight loss forever. Each new day presents changes and challenges. I feel heavier today because of the beer and pizza I enjoyed last night. I remember as I head to breakfast to do my best to make good choices. Then I forget about my tighter "pizza pants" and I forget about my breakfast choices. I know that my daily food choices are now a habit, and I will make them without thinking about it. The subjects of food and my weight are now on the back burner. I have more important things to think about and focus on.

First of all, I enjoy a conversation with my breakfast companions. I learn that Sister Mary Ellen, a retired theology professor, used to check out opera scores from the library, and play and sing things from them with her siblings—like the quartet from *Rigoletto*—and she proceeds to sing a few lines in Italian from that selection. We sing together a phrase or two of the "Habanera" from the opera *Carmen*. Another sister comments that she didn't know she was coming to breakfast for such entertainment. Sister Mary Ellen and a fellow sister purchased standing-room tickets for Wagner's opera *Lohengrin*. I talk of having purchased four-dollar student tickets complete with desks and lights in the top ring of the Metropolitan Opera when I was a student.

What delightful shared experiences I'm learning about, and from these new people in my life. I am in the moment. My weight and what I eat are not on my mind. Back at home in the morning with family, I might hear about my husband's plans for his day, how he feels at the breakfast table. Sitting with family in the morning, I may answer my children's questions. And so my day will proceed. There is no time or energy to focus on my weight. There is too much to be done to spend my time focused on a self-involved topic such as my weight. However, if in the process of creating a new habit you care to make healthy breakfast choices, then of course this will require concentration and focus. The only way to create a habit is to repeat a thought and/or an action over and over *with* focus until it becomes a habit. Then the habit is just that, a program running in the background, just as one computer program runs in the background while we work on another. We work at making a change. We look forward to the change just as we look forward to the change in the weather.

In the second instance, the reacquaintance with an old friend, she and I take great joy in the moment of recognition. We immediately forget about the physical changes we see. In my moment of friend recognition this morning, I think instantly of the camping trip we took together along with Sister Mary Alma about 45 years ago. We were all sisters at the time. Now the other two remain sisters, while I long ago left the convent. In this case, change isn't given a thought. The reconnection of two friends is front and center. I see a few more wrinkles and a few extra pounds, but that doesn't matter. True friends accept each other as they are. This is why the desire to lose weight and keep it off must come from within. Those who love you, love you the way you are. I believe in a God who loves me the way I am, fat or thin. The loss of weight is a welcome change but not a required change for friendship. No one can create a lifetime habit to please another. You must develop weight-loss and maintenance habits for *you*. Your friends will applaud.

In the third instance, making technology changes is very much like making weight-loss changes. Some of us accept the changes and make them; others change kicking and screaming for external reasons—for instance, your job requires it and you don't want to be fired. Many of us just don't change, and become frozen forever in time. I entered the convent at a time of great change in the Catholic Church, just after Vatican II and the aggiornamento created by Pope John XXIII. Mass was said in English; the altar was turned around to face the people; sisters were exchanging their habits for street clothes. Sisters were leaving the convent in droves.

It was also a time of big changes in the kitchen and in the eating habits of the nuns. Sister Grace Ann, a registered dietitian, was now in charge of the kitchen. The old days of snacking on jelly bread while doing the laundry in the morning and indulging in plates of chocolates in the afternoon were over. (All gifts, like boxes of chocolate candy, were turned in, later to be shared by everyone.) No more forced membership in the "clean-plate club." With Sister Grace Ann we were served balanced meals of average proportions, and no one was forced to eat anything. The stage was set for me to lose 50 pounds in the convent.

NUTRITION FOR THE SOUL

In a book with the word "diet," you'd assume that somewhere the concepts of good nutrition would appear. This is not a scientific discussion of food, though it is a book about common-sense food habits.

This morning I reflect more philosophically about the word "nutrition." Here at the convent I head to the dining room three times a day for meals, and I assume that I am receiving good nutrition and won't get fat. "It ain't necessarily so," as Porgy sings in the opera *Porgy and Bess*. The meals are served buffet style, as mentioned, and I have choices to make. On the same buffet, I have a choice of beef burgundy with noodles or baked chicken; French fries or baked sweet potatoes. Which entrée and side are the better choices for weight loss and weight-loss maintenance? And if I can't decide, there is no mother superior standing over me to keep me from taking all four entrées and sides. In the beginning of a weight-loss program, you must learn about which are the best choices. Then you must consciously practice making those choices so they become a habit. Finally here I've created my habit, and I am able to go through the buffet line, chatting with friends, and without thought I choose baked chicken and baked sweet potatoes.

I'm here in the convent, but the days of having the choices made for me are gone. Maybe it's no accident that there is a Weight Watchers meeting held here weekly in Conception Abbey Hall? My food "honeymoon" here is over. At first it was great fun to take some of everything, and how could I resist the nightly array of homemade cookies? Now I know those cookies or homemade bars will be there every day, and I take them only sometimes—and I take one cookie, not two cookies...or four or five cookies.

The real nutrition I am receiving here is that of friendship, with conversation running from "getting to know you" to in-depth sharing of core values and philosophy of life. I have many moments of silence and time for reflection, which is nutrition for my soul and spirit. I have time for reading, which provides necessary nutrients for personal growth. And finally, or in my personal view firstly, I have time for liturgy and spiritual direction. Tonight I will attend the centering prayer group, which helps keep my life on track and keeps me centered as a person. If I forget to attend or make other plans for that time period, there is no reprimand. Centering prayer is just an entrée on the platter of spiritual nutrition offered here in the convent. I am not here for a lifetime but for only a few weeks. I try to be a pig and choose as many spiritual entrées from the platter as I can digest.

Focusing on being centered as a person makes it a lot easier to pass up the French fries.

When I return home, I will again prepare my own meals. I will also remember to create a platter of spiritual entrées for myself to go with those meals...and pass up the French fries.

CHOICES YOU CAN MAKE

Yesterday was a day out of the ordinary at the convent. Many of us went to the local concert hall, a renovated gingerbread jewel of a theater, intimate by design, to hear the Dubuque Symphony. From my front-row center-balcony seat, I felt suspended above the audience below, just in front of the stage. The religious community of sisters owns a subscription of four seats, which are raffled off before each concert. In addition, many of the sisters have their own personal subscription, so the nuns were there by the carload. All the baroque plastered curves and ornate decorations provided the perfect acoustic setting—many surfaces to bounce the sound around the hall. The first notes sent relaxing breaths and shivers pulsating through my body. I enjoyed an afternoon of musical meditation.

I arrived home (the convent, which is my home right now) just in time for happy hour. Happy hour occurs on the last Sunday of the month. Tables were set with an array of drink selections: liqueurs, wine, hard liquor, and soda. A very capable sister dressed in a decorated navy sweatshirt, with a smiling face and a head of beautiful white hair, mixed the drinks. The sister next to me ordered a gin martini. I settled for a glass of red wine. Next I grazed the hors d'oeuvres table and selected slices of hot sausage, veggie pizza, and some sort of cheese bread topped with cooked onions, all worth going back for seconds. The portions were very small, I said to myself, so why not?

I sat at a table near to and with a direct view of the bar. To my amazement, I saw only one sister come back for a second glass of wine. Shortly after, the bartender disappeared. No one returned to the table to help herself to a drink.

I sat alone at the table after my rather raucous four tablemates went off to play cards or to tend to undisclosed personal matters. I just looked around the room at all the beaming faces and animated conversations. Supper was announced, which was eaten by some. I left the room to put on my running shoes for a walk around the building's corridors, as it was a rainy, blustery day. What a delightful infusion of warmth (double entendre intended) the cocktail hour provided on such a cold day.

CREATING SPACE

It has been raining all day. I've learned to eat dinner a little later than the scheduled 5:30 suppertime here at the convent. I select a few cold cuts and salad, and yes, dessert from the buffet table, and take my tray upstairs to the kitchenette near my room to eat later.

I've returned to a "secret little place" that probably everyone knows about but that is not often used. It's a little closed-in porch in the old motherhouse behind a set of stairs. This used to be an open set of stairs with a landing. The stairs are gone and the landing is now a closed-in porch. It's just big enough for four comfortable chairs and a small end table. On the table sits a small flower arrangement, a short pencil, and what looks like a score sheet from a long-finished card game. This is where I set my bottle of water and bag of chips (yes, that's a bag of Cheetos I'm eating). There's a fan with lights suspended from the ceiling. I turn on the light and settle into the comfortable chair from which I will have the best view of the grounds, and open my book. I listen to the rain pounding on the roof above me. I feel suspended in nature as I look out two floor-to-ceiling windows. I feel cozy in my wool sweater. The rain won't get me wet, and its constant patter soothes my spirit. I see so much green. Am I really in Ireland? Seems like it, as I am used to the Southern California desert landscape that normally surrounds me.

Finally I begin reading my book, written by a former student of Sister Mary St. Clara, whose recipes are contained in this book. It's fun to read about "The Kitchen of Tomorrow" as it was presented in 1944. I am not only suspended in nature; I am suspended in time. This motherhouse was built in 1892. There are so many winding paths, turrets, and hidden spaces that I feel like I'm lost in a magic castle…a magic holy castle, perhaps.

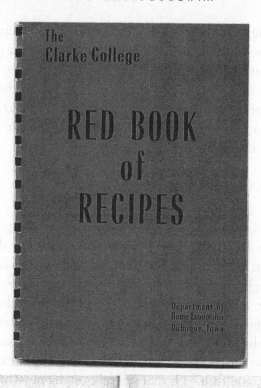

The
Clarke College

RED BOOK
of
RECIPES

Department of
Home Economics
Dubuque, Iowa

HOW TO FOLLOW THE RECIPES

1. Use standard measuring cups and spoons.
2. Use level measurements.
3. Sift flour once before measuring (in baking recipes).
4. Recipes are made with all-purpose flour unless otherwise stated.
5. The size and shape of your baking pan often affects the quality of your finished product. When you have determined which of your pans is the right size, note it on your recipe.

* * * *

HOW TO MEASURE

1. Use one cup to measure all ingredients. Measure dry ingredients first; then fats; then syrups.
2. Measure flour after it has been sifted once.
3. Use two pieces of paper when sifting flour. Sift from one paper to the other.
4. Brown sugar must be firmly packed in the cup to be measured.

* * * *

TABLE OF WEIGHTS AND MEASURES

3 teaspoons	1 tablespoon
4 tablespoons	one-fourth cup
16 tablespoons	1 cup
1 cup	one-half pint
1 cup	8 fluid ounces
2 pints	1 quart
4 quarts	1 gallon
4 pecks	1 bushel
16 ounces	1 pound

9

SOME GENERAL RULES FOR MENU PLANNING

PLAN:

1. The whole day as a unit rather than as three separate meals.

2. The breakfast first and then the dinner.

3. The luncheon or supper so as to supplement the other two meals, and to utilize left-overs.

4. To have in every meal *one* food at least, which has high satiety value—staying quality; one food which requires chewing; one which contains roughage, and generally, even in summer, some hot food or drink.

5. To include in your menus, bland foods and those of more pronounced flavor.

6. For variety in form, color and arrangement.

7. The use of foods crisp in texture as well as soft foods.

8. To avoid too much of any one foodstuff in the menu, such as too much starch, too much fat, or too much protein.

9. For surprises in the meals, to avoid monotony in recipes, color, and seasoning.

10. To combine simple and less nutritious foods with those which are more nutritious and richer in quality.

11. For variety, but not at the expense of food essentials.

12. To avoid serving the same food twice in the same meal, even in different forms.

13. To serve fewer rich foods in small portions, when a number of foods are prepared.

14. To serve larger portions of a few nutritious foods, if a more simple meal is desired.

14

Red Book of Recipes, published 1944

I'm in a time warp. Much is the same, yet much has changed. I embrace the change as a relished memory of the past, and live in the present. I can create my own future, having learned many lessons here in the past. I remember what it felt like to be overweight and how I learned in the novitiate to feel good about myself. I see myself walking into the future as an everyday type of thin person, not a fashion model. I create space inside of me to be at peace with who I am, inside and out.

POSITIVE SELF-TALK

Every morning I read a short meditation and a short inspirational message. My goal is to point my day in a positive and productive direction. Today I think as I reflect: Meditation is a kind of self-talk. We run conversations with ourselves through our heads every day on an ongoing basis. That self-talk can be positive. For example, "Today I'm going to tackle that challenging project on my plate and I'm going to finish it," or, "Today, I'm going to be more open and helpful to my husband when he asks me to show him how to do something on the computer," or, "Today I'm going to eat a good breakfast of egg, oatmeal, and fruit." Or that self-talk can be negative. Using the same three examples, negative self-talk might sound like this: "That project on my plate is so impossible, I don't think I'll even try to work on it today," or, "My husband is always interrupting me and I can't get anything done," or, "That homemade cinnamon bread will just get stale if I don't eat it, so I'll have a slice with butter and skip the oatmeal and fruit. I can't lose weight anyway. I've tried to diet three times and always gained the weight right back."

Today I will indulge in only positive self-talk.

LIVING IN THE MOMENT

I opened my drapes this morning expecting to see either a sunny or cloudy, maybe cloudy and rainy, day. Much to my surprise, as I pulled back the drapes, fog engulfed my world outside. I was delighted to see something I wasn't expecting, something different. I stood in front of the window gazing out for a few moments, taking in the scene in detail. What does that tree, covered with white blossoms just two weeks ago, look like today? Are there any birds flying through the fog? I walked away from the window and headed to the kitchen to make my morning coffee. When I returned to the window, the fog had disappeared. The early morning often brings views that last only a moment. I checked the weather forecast on my phone for tomorrow, vowing to get up in time to see the sun rise over the Mississippi River.

In life, sometimes we see things in black or white, sunny or cloudy. Yet often the joy is in the diversity. How boring it would be if only two species of flowers bloomed in spring: daffodils and tulips, say. I would have to go through life without smelling the lilacs or watching a tiny lily of the valley gradually open, sights I enjoy each day when I'm out for my walk. I remember vividly from one of my philosophy classes in college a quote from the book *The Ethics of Ambiguity*, by Simone de Beauvoir, existentialist and longtime lover of Jean-Paul Sartre: "The degree to which we have a tolerance for ambiguity is the degree to which we are a mature person." There are simple ambiguities in life; for example, "Is that wall paint gray or taupe?" In a moment, we see the black-and-white answer by turning on a light. Ambiguity in the world of intangibles can be more frustrating. For example, "Will I truly achieve permanent weight loss?" I'm doing everything I can to reach my goal, but will it happen? I must live my life in the ambiguity of not knowing the answer to that question.

During the beginning days of dieting we are most anxious to see results. "I want to lose 50 pounds, and today I'm down one pound. What will the scale say tomorrow?" We must live with the process, knowing that we are taking the steps necessary to accomplish our goal. The hard part is the process itself, the waiting in ambiguity. Just as I pull the drapes to check out the day's weather, I get on the scale each morning to check out my weight and stay the course.

I accept the process and live in the moment.

TOMORROW IS ANOTHER DAY

I set my alarm last night for 5:45 a.m., as the sun was expected to rise today at 5:53 a.m. I went to sleep with great expectations of viewing a beautiful sunrise in the morning. I thought back on the many trips to Hawaii I had taken with my mother. We always stayed in the same room in the same hotel. We did this for about 30 years—just the two of us, none of my brothers allowed. From our room, we had a spectacular view of the sunrise. It was different every day but always worth getting up early to see.

The alarm rang this morning and I hit the snooze button. However, the desire to see the sunrise overtook the urge to continue sleeping, and I got up and opened the drapes. There is an eastern view from my room if one looks left, but the view is primarily a southern one. I decided I couldn't see enough, so I put on my robe and scurried out the door, heading for one of the turret rooms. I started with the third-floor turret (fewer stairs to climb), arrived there, and looked out the window. A big tree was in the way. I climbed another flight of stairs to the fourth-floor turret. The view there was better, and I knew there was nowhere else to go to improve my view—at least nowhere that wasn't locked or somebody's bedroom. It was cold in the turret but I stuck it out, determined to catch a beautiful sunrise. 15 minutes passed, and the sun peeked through the clouds, looking somewhat attractive but still not the colorful array I had imagined.

Should I try again tomorrow or give up? That big tree will be there again and maybe the sunrise won't be that great anyway. On the other hand, I won't know if there will be a beautiful sunrise tomorrow unless I get up, *again*, run up to the fourth-floor turret, *again*, being sure to grab a sweater as I go out the door, and look. The sound of the train whistle rang out today as the sun came up, just as it is sounding now as I write. This is the self-talk going on in my head. Is trying again worth the effort? Sunrise, or sleep; sunrise, or sleep. Which will it be?

Is this not the dilemma we encounter trying to lose weight and keep it off? We eat correctly all day and run to the scale the next morning with great anticipation, and often we don't see the number we are hoping for on that scale. God forbid after doing everything right we see an even higher number than we saw yesterday on the scale. Do we try again tomorrow, and the next day and the next day? Or do we decide, "Oh well, it's impossible. I'm just destined to be overweight. I give up."

I think again about that sunrise I'm envisioning and dreaming about. Do I try again tomorrow and if I don't see something spectacular, say, "Oh well, there will never be a beautiful sunrise, so I'll just sleep through it every morning and forget about it"? We know that to say there will never be a beautiful sunrise again is a ridiculous statement. Isn't telling ourselves that we can never lose weight just as ridiculous a statement?

AGE IS JUST A NUMBER

How old is old? There is always the saying "You're as young as you feel," or as someone shared with me years ago, "Old is anyone 15 years older than you are now." When I first heard this latter phrase, that would have made "old" about 45 years of age. Today I should be so young!

Today is my tenth wedding anniversary. I opened two cards from my husband before I did anything else except grab a cup of coffee. I thought back on our wedding day as I watched two squirrels scamper under my window as a pair, one plump and one wiry. Were they mates, I wondered? Yesterday, Sister Mary Alma, my high school journalism teacher and lifelong friend, said to me, "I'm a senator [in the congregation]. I'm 87 years old; do you think I should run again for office?" There are many reasons to run or not run for office, but since she prefaced her question with the phrase "I'm 87 years old," I thought she was looking for an answer to the question, "Am I too old?" In a flash, I thought back on my wedding day as a late-in-life bride, of how involved my mother had been in the process of preparing for the wedding. Mother was probably about 87 years old at the time. She flew back and forth from Minnesota to Los Angeles almost monthly before the wedding for dress fittings, reception planning, and food tastings. Planning a wedding with me was something she had been looking forward to for years. Mother seemed ageless to me.

Back to Sister Mary Alma and her question. Sister is my daily consultant, confidante, and advisor as I write this book. How can she be 87? I answered that 87 was not too old *for her* to be a senator if that's what she wanted to do.

And finally this morning I am reflecting on a lunch conversation this week with someone I will call Sister Therese, who was clearly overweight and probably also in her eighties. As Sister talked and laughed, I recognized that New York Italian accent. As the conversation continued, I imagined I was talking to one of my Italian husband's sisters. My new friend had heard through the convent grapevine that I was writing a "diet" book. She peppered me with questions about what she should do to lose weight. I heard long explanations of all the things she had tried and been advised to do, including attending Weight Watchers, which was to date her most successful effort. Sister had lost 20 pounds but gained back ten pounds. She went on to discuss exercise. I heard all the things she "should" do, none of which she did. Then the reasons and excuses followed. I heard the usual things along with several health conditions that sounded serious.

We often expect the elderly not to worry about weight. We believe they think, "At this age, why should I worry about diet?" Here was an elderly sister with serious health issues who hadn't given up the ghost; she wanted to lose weight. If I closed my eyes, I would think I was listening to someone about 50 years old trying to get rid of middle-aged spread. Two of the many things I said brought a smile to Sister's face: First, "Think of one thing you're going to do today toward your weight-loss goals, such as yogurt for breakfast, and then forget about it. Focus on what's important to you today—what you are going to read, the class you will attend, and the friends you will chat with—but eat that yogurt."

Anytime I'm tempted to think I should accept extra weight gain because I'm older now or that doing something I enjoy that takes a little physical activity should be skipped today, I just think of Sister Therese.

At any age, it can be tempting to think: 1) "I've carried these extra 20 pounds around for the last ten or 20 years, so I'll just accept being over-weight" and 2) "I don't have time to play the piano today." Turn those state-ments around: 1) "I've carried around 20 extra pounds for 20 years, and today will be the first day of the rest of my life without them" and 2) "I'm going to play the piano for half an hour after dinner tonight, maybe even before I do the dishes."

POSITIVE ENERGY

Being surrounded by good people is like living in a beautiful garden. Good people create a peace and calmness around us, as if we're smelling lilacs and gazing on a sea of multicolored rosebushes. Each rose is unique not just in color but in shape and size. All are beautiful.

What a joy it is for me to be here at the convent surrounded by so many beautiful faces, warm smiles, and kind gestures. Each day I go to the dining room for a meal and wonder whom I will meet and what stories they will share. Or I go down knowing with whom I will sit because we have much to discuss.

Good people are buoyant; they lift those around them. I still join the centering prayer group once a week, but every day I am inspired to do things and just be my best me because of the good people surrounding me. Good people give me energy. I am inspired by those who wear a smile but are in constant pain. If the Sisters can bring good energy to their day and to those around them, I can do it too, whether I'm in physical pain or experiencing the agony of a nagging problem.

This positive energy helps me keep on track for the day. I am infused with enthusiasm to begin the tasks of my day, to continue them, to march onward. With this energy, I can keep on track with my food choices because there is the food of friendship at the table to help me out.

If I am not surrounded by good people, then it's up to me to make a change. While change can be scary and painful, coming out on the other side of change feels ebullient. I want to make the good habits I've created as easy as possible to follow. I'm the only one who can do that.

GO WITH THE FLOW

The window washers were here yesterday in the early morning, just in time to interrupt my reflections for the day. Then the phone began ringing and seemed not to stop. Phone calls take me off track in different directions. Each call generally requires some action on my part as a follow-up, and there goes my day, down the yellow brick road to Oz.

I was determined not to let distractions set the tone for my day. Frustration and/or anger set a tone of negativity for the rest of the day. I was also determined not to grieve for the loss of time. That was the hardest part.

I managed to go with the flow, as they say. I did what I could do and moved on. The approach didn't bring back the time, but it brought acceptance.

Today I am benefiting from the clean windows. The view is so clear; yesterday's window washers helped make today special. Sometimes it works that way. My early-morning time today was especially productive.

How many times do we say to ourselves something like, "I just ate a pizza for supper followed by a whole box of Thin Mints Girl Scout cookies, eaten one by one while watching the news after dinner. I didn't even realize I ate the whole box. I give up. I'll never lose weight."

This happens. The pizza and cookies were the window washers that stole your good intentions. Tomorrow is a new day. It is the first day of the rest of your life. Tomorrow is day one. Forget about yesterday. Things always look better in the morning after a good night's sleep anyway.

The key is that I am not on a diet. I am living my life. This is day one of the rest of my life, so I have plenty of time to begin again. What will I do differently today so it is not a repeat of yesterday? The cookies are gone now; I won't buy any more and the cupboard is clean. The window washers are gone, leaving behind a clean slate.

Today I'll have a piece of lemon Bundt cake that I stored in the freezer in slices. I'll thaw only one slice to eat while I watch the news tonight.

TAKING TIME TO SHARE

We all know the old saying "Don't judge a book by its cover." I learned that lesson anew yesterday at lunch. I sat with Sister May and Sister Edna, but Sister Edna left promptly to go to an appointment. Sister May and I spent almost the next hour talking, just the two of us. I had seen Sister May around but had not met her. Sister was elderly and frail-looking, bent, had almost no hair, and always wore what appeared to be a white neck brace or large bandage. She spoke in a scratchy whisper.

Sister told me that she came here from the South. I don't meet many from the South, so I was immediately curious about her story. Sister's roots are really in Chicago's South Side Italian community. With this disclosure, we immediately bonded, because I'm married to an Italian from New York whose immigrant parents married in Positano, Italy, before coming to this country. Sister worked primarily in the South with the African American community throughout her teaching career. I heard tales of tragedy and prejudice and through it all, I heard one sister's tale of joy. I heard about how much Sister misses her mission, but it's clear that Sister now needs help herself.

The dining room quieted as many sisters finished their lunches and left. Then we got down to the core of the story. Sister suffers from an autoimmune disease (scleroderma) that is clearly life-threatening. Sister May said, "There is no cure for this disease; I am going to die." She added that she is not afraid of death. But what I heard next was shocking to me: "Some days I don't believe in God. Other days the feelings of God's presence around me are overpowering." She isn't sure about Jesus, she stated matter-of-factly. I was reminded of my many financial planning interviews throughout my 30-year practice as a financial advisor. I have heard many shocking stories and personal views, which I always accepted as if I were on the same page with the client, to allow that person to continue without fear of judgment. Only in truth can there be true sharing. Only in truth can people truly help each other. I proceeded to share my own feelings and doubts with Sister. She listened and nodded her head in agreement.

I sensed that it probably was time to attend Sister Diane's final children's music program in the next building. Sister Diane is retiring from her long career as a grammar school music teacher. I have known her since our novitiate days over 50 years ago, so I wanted to be there. Sister May and I walked over together as if hand in hand. I don't know the rest of Sister May's name, but I have shared thoughts from her heart and soul. How could I have overlooked her these past few weeks to sit down to lunch with others who were perhaps younger and seemingly more vibrant? No one here is more alive than Sister May.

DIVERSITY OF THOUGHT

I've been back here at the convent for a month now, and I am struck by all the changes that I see have happened since I lived here as well as all the diversity among the sisters. Most important, I see a great acceptance of that diversity. This is not the old days. This is the way to real personal growth and understanding and acceptance of each self. Yet I believe these habits of growth, understanding, and acceptance were envisioned by my novice mistress for all of her charges over 50 years ago. I know this because this is what I got out of her instruction each morning those many years ago. Sister embraced change and led us in that direction. The mother superior at the time must have approved. Our novice mistress never heard, "You're fired." However, as mentioned, that was a time of great turbulence in the Catholic Church following the conclusion of Vatican II in 1962. Pope John XXIII opened the doors and let in some fresh air. He turned the altar around and communicated with his people instead of preaching at them. What was begun here at the convent over 50 years ago has now come to fruition. Sisters claim their careers of choice. This is no longer a teaching order. I am not a fallen-away nun or an ex-nun; I am an associate in the order who is most welcome. I live here now among the sisters as if I am one of them. No space is off-limits, and I am excluded from nothing. I see just now a sister walking out the door of the building next to this one. She is wearing a veil. Most in this community do not wear the veil, but the choice of dress here is personal. Sisters from other communities are also welcome, veil or no veil. Finally, there is the same diversity now, here behind the convent wall, that has been on the grounds in front of the convent wall since forever.

I wake up each morning, look out my window, and see in front of the convent something different every day. No tree is the same, even among a single species. One tree caught my eye this morning as the sun beamed through it, creating a shimmering translucence. The tree is no longer transparent, as it was a month ago when its limbs were bare. The multiple shades of green contrast with the limbs and branches, at this moment colored black by the sun's shadows.

As I sit here and write about my weight-loss experiences behind the convent wall, sharing these experiences, hoping they will help others, I think about the diversity in diets because of the diversity in people. There are as many diets as there are people, which is as it should be. If one thought I share from the convent helps one person, my work will have been accomplished. I relish the diversity and take my place within it.

PLOWING AHEAD

The tops of the trees were really swaying this morning. I'm wondering how windy it will feel outside today. I decide to think about going out in the wind later and watching the birds flying in and out of the big tree in front of my window. So many are so colorful. I focus on what I think at first glance is a robin because of the red in its breast area. Then I notice a bit of yellow and know it must be some other bird. My yellow-and-red friend clings to one of the top tree branches and sways back and forth. It's so tiny and the wind so strong; how does this bird cling to the branch? Is it difficult to cling, or is it just habit?

Sometimes my life seems so combative, I feel like I'm walking through a wind tunnel. I keep walking despite the headwinds pushing me back. Do I deliberately choose to keep walking, or is it just habit to plow ahead in life? For me, I think the answer is a little of each. I wake up each day planning to move forward, though each day there are setbacks to battle. Sometimes I can't plow ahead purely out of habit. I must make a mindful and deliberate decision to keep going.

Even the most enjoyable of jobs has its nitty-gritty moments. Does that mean it's time for a new job? Not to me. It just means I need to handle the nitty-gritty knowing that doing so will be worth it. I practice the piano daily, struggling with a particularly difficult passage until I can play it smoothly. I go for a walk every day even though it's windy or a bit too cold or a bit too hot.

Every day I follow the Seven Holy Habits to keep my weight in check. Some days the habits are easy; I'm on autopilot and I don't think about them really. Some days I struggle. I couldn't resist the second, third, or fourth slice of pizza. I move on. Tomorrow is a new day. Maybe the headwinds won't be so strong.

ACCEPTANCE

Today I felt like a hidden guest at a dinner party as I looked out from my window. My view includes another wing of this building, the beautiful stained glass windowed entrance with offices extending on the bottom and bedrooms above. Attached is a large patio, almost a balcony, as it sits up half a flight of stairs adjoining the stately entrance. A bird feeder is attached to one of the office windows by a suction cup. A little chickadee pecks at dinner in the feeder. Below scurries a chipmunk, licking the leftovers, and a large mourning dove bobs along, sharing the feast with the chipmunk. A beautiful blue jay flies in, lands on the patio railing, and just watches. The blue jay flies again and lands right under my window, closes its wings, and displays its full body coloration, glistening in the sun. I wait for the blue jay to bully the other birds away, as I've heard that is the blue jay's nature, but this doesn't happen. Here I watch birds large, medium, and small plus a lowly rodent sharing at the table. Above soars a crow, paying no mind to what is going on below. The rumble of a distant train blowing its horn bothers no bird.

If only people could be more like the birds and chipmunk, sharing at the table of life, delighting in diversity. People don't live by instinct alone, however. We lead with our emotions. We talk about the importance of making rational decisions. I often think our decisions are made with emotions. We use rationalization to back up our emotional decisions.

This emotion-reason conflict carries through to every aspect of life. Specifically, I now think about diversity of size and weight. Eating too much for many of us is tied to emotions. Restaurants even have "comfort foods," including things like macaroni and cheese and mashed potatoes and gravy. I crave macaroni and cheese after a hard day. If I have a 14-ounce box of macaroni and cheese in the cupboard, I make it and eat the whole thing myself.

The heavier I get, the unhappier I become. People around me seem to favor the thinner women, just like in grade school. I was the heaviest child in the class and the last one picked for the ball team by my team captain peer, and the last one chosen by my third-grade teacher, Sister Roselima, to stay after school and clean the blackboards. The latter was not a chore but a privilege; the blackboard cleaner was the chosen one.

Where does this end? For me it ended in the convent, where I was accepted for who I was, not for what I looked like. Later, after I left the convent and headed for Broadway hoping to make it to the stage, I dated an older man briefly who owned a chain of Middle Eastern restaurants. His name was Nathan Steinman. He said, "You don't behave like a typical beautiful woman. You don't trade on your looks." My life is not about my looks. While the world around me judges people based on looks, I was lucky enough to spend a period of time in my most formative years in a place where looks didn't matter. Once I believed in my acceptance as me, I was able to focus on things other than food. I found comfort elsewhere, starting with the comfort of knowing, being, and accepting who I was and am. Self-acceptance is the beginning of permanent weight loss.

WHY I LEFT THE CONVENT

I guess the Peggy Lee song "Is That All There Is?" tells part of my story. I thought I was happy in the convent. I was surrounded by seemingly happy and well-adjusted sisters, inspiring in their devotion to their mission and to God. Community life felt comfortable to me. The sisters valued education and each other. I loved the ordered life we led.

I didn't think about leaving until Father Rulla suggested that I felt my life was empty. Who, you may ask, is Father Rulla? Father Luigi Rulla is a psychiatrist. The mother superior allowed him to study three groups of young sisters in formation, testing to find the reasons for entering and leaving religious life as research for a book he was writing with Joyce Ridick and Franco Imoda: *Entering and Leaving Vocation: Intrapsychic Dynamics* (Gregorian & Biblical Press, 1976). I was in Group C, the last of the three groups. Every six months or so we were given a battery of tests, including the Minnesota Multiphasic Personality Inventory test (with all the sex questions blacked out, of course). I don't recall the number of years during which we were tested. After a time, anyone who desired could meet with Father Rulla to learn the results of her tests personally. I did so and remember being told I felt my life was empty. I gave this sentence much thought and determined that Father Rulla was in a way correct. I had no idea what was missing. Is that the definition of empty?...not knowing what, if anything, is missing?

I did not leave right away, but could not stop thinking about what was missing in my life. The discomfort over the question is why I left the convent. It was only years later, looking back, that I could more fully answer.

Leaving was about curiosity and career.

Maybe the empty feeling had to do with wondering about all the things I had given up without ever having experienced them. I had never really dated, though I did manage to go to the prom in high school. I went to an all-girls school, so in that pre–women's lib era, the girls would ask the boys to the prom. I can't believe Mike, the boy I asked, said yes. Unbeknownst to me, until Mike showed up at my mother's wake in 2015, did I learn that Mike considered himself to be a total geek in high school. Was this the prom match of the geek and the overweight teen? I was simply thrilled that Mike said yes, and did not consider him to be a geek. Mike was smart in school and I admired that.

It wasn't about sex; it was about relationships. However, in time, the sex went along with finding new relationships. So a first proposal of marriage at about age 26 satisfied my curiosity. My parents were pleased, though in the end the wedding was not to be.

This was the 1970s; Kent State and Vietnam were the talk of the campus. (I went back to college to finish my degree after leaving the convent.) Gloria Steinem and Phyllis Schlafly were duking it out over equal rights, and I rooted for Steinem. I subscribed to *Ms.* magazine as soon as it was born. I didn't consciously choose career over marriage. I believed you could have it all. I just wanted to get some sort of career established first, to find my own identity.

I became a Certified Financial Planner (CFP) after spending a few years in New York trying my hand at auditioning for operas and Broadway productions, neither a real career choice for women in the 1960s. I've worked in the financial services industry for more than 30 years and am a practicing CFP to this day.

I had entered a teaching order of nuns. As a music major, I just assumed I would be a music teacher or professor. In high school in my day, if you were on the college track, you became either a teacher or a nurse. I knew I didn't want to be a nurse, so I guess I wanted to be a teacher. I had made a choice by default. I never thought there could be other career choices out there for me. As a music teacher in the convent, I wasn't really in the right career.

Looking back, I ask this question: If I had waited to enter the convent until I had had some life experience, and if the order of nuns had accepted all professions as they began doing not many years after I left, would I have left the convent? I think perhaps the answer would be no.

I left for curiosity and career, which, as the years have passed, have become no reason at all. "Is that all there is?" would not be a question.

WEATHERING THE STORM

I wake up today to see the morning after a storm. A storm watch was issued last night, and we all closed our shutters, blinds, and drapes. Out walking in the early evening, I could smell a storm coming without hearing a weather report. The sticky humidity made the air heavy; the slight inclines along my route became a chore. As the sky turned gray and the clouds thickened, I wondered if I would make it back to the convent before the storm. I did indeed reach my room without feeling a drop of rain. I showered away the damp sweat seeping through my T-shirt and watched...

The winds picked up, and indeed the rain poured down in sheets. I worried about the table, chairs, and umbrella set up on the patio below my room, but the wind seemed miraculously to skirt around the patio, keeping safe even the umbrella as well as the glass office windows in the path of flying furniture.

How often I have endured in the eye of a storm of activity, a storm of words, or a storm of life-changing events in which the worst of the winds and rain passed me by. I weathered the storm, as the saying goes.

There is always a morning after, whether sunny or still cloudy and forbidding. Sometimes the storms we experience do not end overnight. The morning sky still threatens. Maybe the storm continues. Yet storms eventually end or move on. Some leave behind only sunshine, while others leave minor or major destruction. How joyous the sunshine even if there is cleanup to do.

Lifelong weight maintenance brings its own storms to weather. Sometimes they are of our own making, and sometimes they can't be helped. Embrace the storm and move on. Do not feel guilty if it was of your own creation.

Begin the morning after with the fresh eyes of a new day. Clean up if necessary and move on.

RENEWAL

Every morning I open my drapes to see the turrets of the convent's motherhouse. My room sits in the jutting arm of a more contemporary building on the campus facing this grand dame of structures. The earlier I rise, the more fascinating the view. One morning the red brick structure featuring arches and turrets was almost hidden by fog. Gradually the turrets and everything attached to them emerged like Brigadoon did. (As the story goes, Brigadoon emerged out of the mist every 100 years.) I live in my own Brigadoon every day. It's called the convent.

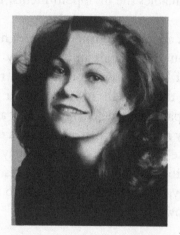

Mary Lou in her first professional headshot, taken shortly after arriving in New York to try her hand at New York music and theatre auditions a few years after leaving the convent. Photo by Christian Steiner.

When I was in the theater in New York, *Brigadoon* was a musical I toured with and performed in many times. Eight times a week I was a citizen of Brigadoon, singing and dancing. I feel I'm still a citizen of Brigadoon now, singing again both literally and from my soul. Only this Brigadoon, the convent, is here every day and has been here since 1892. I call it "the magic castle" because there are so many hidden rooms, nooks, and crannies. I referred to the motherhouse structure as the magic castle to one of my sister friends one day, and she said, "It's the *holy* magic castle." I don't think it's holy, but

I didn't disagree with Sister. This motherhouse tells decidedly human stories of some very holy and yes, not so holy, women. But then, who am I to judge who is holy? I showed Sister, who has lived here for two years, the way to a small room on the fourth floor behind an unmarked door; it's a room large enough for only two glider rockers and a small end table sitting in front of floor-to-ceiling windows. The windows revealed a bird's-eye view of rolling hills and trees, a patchwork of many shades of green. These for me were windows to the world of the Midwest.

I come up here to read, meditate, and reach out to nature. I register what I see; I'm not rushing around in my usual way. I reflect on the mundane as well as the abstract. There is a place for all thoughts and feelings. I feel safe up here, maybe even safe from myself and my world of "I should...." This is a place of renewal, a place to find the courage again to live my life. I can even think about the unthinkable: the disappointments, the betrayals, and other painful things.

I even dare to think about my journey with weight control—or not. I can face the past pain not out of nostalgia and negativity. I say, "What can I learn from the experience of being heavy, and how can this propel me into the future?" Remembering the pain tells me that I never want to be heavy again. Contemplation of the pain gives me energy to meet another day focused and in control. I don't really need to eat half a chicken; a quarter of a chicken will do, because I see a piece of chocolate cake in my day today.

This is only a fleeting thought of food. I am resolute in my purpose for today. I hop on the elevator and head downstairs to the dining room with a smile, centered in my own strength.

WEARING YOUR BEST FACE

Since I have been staying here at the convent, scaffolding has been set up and gradually moved around the facade of the old motherhouse. Masons are tuck-pointing the brick. This week the artisans are working on the front section of the building in full view from my window. I stand and watch for a moment each morning. How tedious is this job, yet how very important. Incorrectly done tuck-pointing can cause irreparable damage. Knife in one hand and trowel in the other hand, the mason carefully pushes new mortar between each brick, careful to match the old and the new. Old, cracked mortar and dust have been cleaned away. This 1892 motherhouse is a state landmark building, and it's getting a face-lift.

I put on a little makeup this morning and think about how I put on a new face each morning before I go out to meet the sisters. Before I apply the makeup, I'm careful to clean my face. Layering makeup on a dirty face or layering new makeup on top of old makeup will only cause damage to my skin. At age 69, I don't really worry about the wrinkles or try to cover them up with foundation, but I do care about the health of my skin, the largest organ of the body. A clean face is a fresh face. The motherhouse is looking more vibrant each day. The tuck-pointing will never make it look new again, or even as new as the 1960s building I'm calling home while here. My fresh face, even with a bit of makeup added, will never make me look as young as my beautiful daughters-in-law, but I will be wearing my best face. I will never again be as young as I am today. As I have learned from the nuns around me, the best and most youthful thing I can put on my face is not a bit of makeup but a big smile.

My fresh face, complete with smile, makes me beautiful no matter the perfection and age of my features, no matter the perfection and age of my body. As I begin each day, practicing my habits to lose weight and keep it off, I know that my smile makes me beautiful and ageless. My smile makes extra pounds invisible to others. I visualize a beautiful me. I present to others the beauty that is inside of me. Extra pounds are not first and foremost. I focus on saying mentally to each person I meet, "How can I help?" while in the background, weight-loss strategies are growing into habits. The pounds will come off and stay off in good time.

AVAILABILITY AND OPTIONS

It felt strange to see a group of sisters in habits going through the breakfast buffet line this morning, some in white veils (novices) and some in black veils (professed sisters). Judging from the long brown garb and rope belt, I would say they were Franciscans. Almost no one wears a habit anymore in the order I was a part of. The few who do are in the infirmary and are generally quite elderly. Sister Marian asked me yesterday if I had seen a group of sisters in habits. I had seen the group in front of the infirmary and said so. That seemed to heighten Sister's expectation. As the Bob Dylan song that I sang so often with my guitar in the novitiate goes, the times they are a-changin'. I thought nothing of seeing habited sisters in or around the infirmary, because as one of the larger orders, ours takes care of seriously ill sisters from other smaller communities who do not have our facilities. The cloistered Trappistines, also in habits, have had sisters here recently, for example.

This morning, I stood over the trays of fresh donuts, trying to decide which one to pick, and one of the brown-habited novices asked me which one was best. I told her that every Saturday I make a different donut choice, hoping to try as many different ones as possible, and that "best" was up to her. We discussed cake donuts versus raised donuts and the properties of each. Another sister came by, incredulous that I would be giving advice on donuts. I wonder if the novice ever had the opportunity to eat donuts. I doubt it, so the choice was, I sensed, significant. Sister selected a raised bar-shaped donut with lots of white icing. We have store-bought donuts every Saturday courtesy of a kind donor. And there are always some left over for the noon meal, so fear of not getting one if you're the last to breakfast is not an issue.

Diversity, scarcity, and wealth were all on display here this morning. How easily we walk among those in habits as if they are one with us. Indeed, they are one with us. The habit is only an outer symbol. Inside we are the same. I say "we" because that sameness is not just that the convent is filled with nuns, but that the convent is filled with human beings. I am no longer a nun, but I am one with each and all. This is the same welcoming place that accepted me and others 50 years ago, rich or poor, young or old, fat or thin.

I know what it feels like to be given a store-bought donut only once in a blue moon, so I appreciate the monumental decision that faced this young novice as to which one to pick. The discussion about the donuts was not really one of instruction as to which donut to pick. It was the sharing of delight in the availability and the options. So often we are feeling that the door to options is closed because of the choices we have made in the past. I don't believe that. I am here at once visiting a familiar past but only as it opens a new door to a new future. I was once that novice. I am again that novice, learning and moving forward.

As I shared this donut experience with both a novice from another order and a longtime professed sister from my order, I saw the wealth we have here. Those donuts arrive every Saturday, and maybe some of us take them for granted. Some of us may always choose the same donut, our favorite. I hope

I never lose the enthusiasm of choice and the surprise of the gift not taken for granted.

FOR MY HUSBAND

Dear John,

I woke up early this morning, 5:30 a.m., so I thought I'd jump up, open the drapes and catch the sunrise. The glimmer of light mixed with shadows on the red brick motherhouse swirled, an orangey pink. I looked to my left to see a thin haze of fuchsia along the river behind the trees. It was worth getting up early for this moment. I longed to text a snapshot of this moment to you, John, but didn't want to awaken you so early, two time zones away. I sat in my rocker, thinking of you. I'll be home soon....

[Later]

I look out at the sunset, lights twinkling on the river, calling me out so quickly that I nearly forget my key. I walk for a while, I call you, I talk to you, I long for you...then I sit on a lonely bench with room enough for two and watch a barge push down the river, all lit up in back. I think, "Are all barges shaped like this, so long and seemingly made of so many pieces?" I don't know. It doesn't look like the barges I see in the daytime. Does it matter? Everything matters. That's the joy of life, the excitement to realize that each moment matters. I will miss this view when I go home, but I long for you.

Yet I just made plans to leave again, to say goodbye again. Why do I plan to say goodbye again when I miss you so? Other voices are calling me, calling me to be away—yes, away for us. The evening is so soft and warm, and I long to lie down with you, with your arms around me. Are your arms empty now without me? Will our love be forever changed by this goodbye? I'm sorry to tell you I'll be leaving again. You work for me, you walk for me, as I walk for you to be my best for you. I give you my best me. Lying by your side is the greatest peace I've ever known. Is my goodbye bringing us together with bonds stronger than ever, I wonder?

I languish walking back to the convent, looking back over my shoulder at the lights, the city shapes and the shimmering river. I say goodbye to this idyllic scene to come home to your arms and the warmth of your love.

REFERENCES

REFERENCES

Course Correction/Nip It in the Bud!

f you find yourself suddenly up five to eight pounds without realizing it or knowing why that happened, when you *do* realize it, the following course correction ideas will be helpful. These are questions I ask myself, especially now that I am older and "have no metabolism," as my doctor told me last week!

1. **ACCOUNTABILITY:**
   a) Are you using the accountability checker daily? Is the checker somewhere, like on your refrigerator, where you will see it even if you aren't thinking about looking for it?
   b) Briefly keep track daily of what you are eating and how much of it you are eating to see where you are getting off track. No one can count daily food intake for a lifetime. Just use this technique temporarily for troubleshooting. For example, I'm cooking dinner and there's a box of Wheat Thins left on the kitchen table by my husband yesterday. Every time I walk by the table during dinner preparation, I grab a few crackers because I can't wait for dinner...hmmmm. Instead, while you're preparing a salad for dinner, clean an extra carrot and eat it—"Chomp, chomp," like Bugs Bunny—right away and get those Wheat Thins back in the cupboard. Or, put your dinner salad portion in a bowl right away and eat it while cooking. Calories are the same whether you eat them at the dinner table with your family or eat them while preparing dinner.
   c) If you're up ten pounds or more before you face the music, you may want to get outside help. Too many people feel that out-

side help is a last-ditch effort only for those who are *really* (500 to 100 pounds) overweight. Not so. There are many excellent weight-loss programs out there. Weight Watchers works for those who need the group accountability and socializing. Jenny Craig and NutriSystem help with learning portion control because they each involve prepared food portions. A psychologist and/or dietitian is always helpful. While you may not stay on NutriSystem forever or visit a psychologist weekly for the rest of your life, you may want to get outside help periodically forever to keep good habits in place and avoid "yo-yo" dieting.

2. **YOU'RE THIN UNTIL YOU'RE THIN, AND THE CONCEPT OF VISUALIZATION:**

The mirror is your wake-up call. Put on an outfit now hanging in your closet that fit perfectly a few months ago, a year ago. (We all have such outfits.) If you're catching weight gain early enough, you'll see that the outfit "still fits" but perhaps doesn't look good. Is your stomach sticking out? Too tight to look good all over? Perhaps you didn't even notice the weight gain if your lifestyle involves living in sweats and chasing after small children—or if your lifestyle involves another kind of relaxed dressing rather than a daily corporate suit. In pull-on pants with a blouse, the extra weight doesn't show the way it does in a fitted business dress. The mirror is your reality check, your truth teller. Listen to what that mirror is telling you. Go back to watching portion sizes perhaps, but try on that same outfit at least once a week until it looks good on you. I love clothes and am highly motivated to eat a low-fat packaged dinner for a couple of nights so I look good in my favorite outfits.

3. **ALWAYS EAT DESSERT:**

a) While this is the main strategy I used to stay thin for 50 years, it can have its flaws. How *much* dessert are you eating? Have you gradually gone back to eating half a box of Thin Mint Girl Scout cookies after dinner for dessert? If yes, it will take time to work your way back to eating only a few cookies after dinner. Never try to go cold turkey and eat no cookies. This is too depressing to stick with for a lifetime. Cut back to one quarter of a box each night until that much leaves you feeling full and satisfied before cutting the portion down further. Accept the fact that a little extra time spent at this point reaps a lifetime of rewards.

b) Try eating dessert at only one meal instead of at both lunch and dinner. Most people don't eat dessert for breakfast, but if you're someone who polishes off a plate of scrambled eggs and toast with a big cinnamon roll, then cut back on dessert one meal at a time until you have dessert at only one meal a day. I have found that as I have aged, this has become necessary for me. This was not true when I was in my thirties, forties, and even fifties.

c) Be sure the dessert you eat is something you really love. Don't eat a cup of Jell-O, for example, because it's low in calories. After the Jell-O, you will just move on and eat that piece of chocolate cake anyway. Eat the cake to begin with; a cup of Jell-O on top of the cake may mean an extra 100 hundred calories.

d) Eat an ever-so-slightly-smaller portion. If you order lemon cake during a lunch out at Nordstrom's, eat half of that cake and bring the other half home. If you brought home the big half, try to make it last for two nights' desserts. I ask the waitress to bring a to-go box with the cake, and immediately put the big half in the box before I eat what's on the plate. Out of sight, out of mind. Portion sizes tend to grow just like the amoebas we studied in biology in high school.

e) Watch your snacks. This category of food tends to grow without notice. Say you're really proud of yourself because you bought a bag of baked vegetable chips instead of regular potato chips. *Don't eat that snack out of the bag.* If one serving size is one ounce, 120 calories, get out the sandwich-size baggies, open your six-ounce bag of chips, and immediately divide the chips into one-ounce-per-baggie servings. Chips are so light, it's amazing how many you can eat and still eat only one ounce. I put the little baggies back in the big bag, keep the bag in the cupboard, and pull out one baggie of chips for my snack as desired. That baggie looks like so many chips, I never eat a second baggie of chips. My mind tells me I'm satisfied, and I focus on something else. If you bring the snack to your work desk, you have just quantified (now I sound like the financial planner I am) your snack. When the baggie is empty, you will be involved in your work and won't get up to get more.

f) *Do not try to give up dessert completely!* If you are a dessert lover, never give up dessert. You will only get fat!

4. DON'T COUNT CALORIES, BUT CALORIES COUNT:

a) If you have gradually begun to eat more food, cutting back will feel like deprivation, and negatives can't work for a lifetime. Take a no-brainer approach to cutting back. I also call this the "accidental" approach to cutting back, because someone else is doing the portion control for you. Eat low-fat packaged dinners for a couple of days on and off until you've lost a couple of pounds. This is also a great time saver for a busy person. Eating packaged dinners gives you more hours in the day to be with your kids, do something you love, or complete those back-burner work projects. For the family, bake or buy a roasted chicken and heat up some frozen veggies and so on, depending on your budget. Never let the need to cook for the family be an excuse for gaining weight. Remember the words of Sister Mary John Thomas: "We always have time to do the things we really want to do." I have a husband who won't try much of anything. I can either choose to cook only what he will eat and limit my own food choices, or I can cook two things. I generally choose to do the latter, even though it takes a little more time and effort. I *really* want to eat the things that are right for me, and I *really* want a happy husband.

b) In the short term, hide the Twinkies and Ding Dongs your kids eat so you don't see them and eat them too. Never leave a void in their place. Have your favorite "reasonable" snacks sitting around in the cupboard. I have a basket in the cupboard just for me, in which I keep individual one- or two-ounce baggies of trail mix and/or nuts, Rice Krispies treats, fig bars, and other things I like that add up to around 100 to 150 calories.

5. AVOID DIET FOOD:

Avoid the temptation to fill up on large volumes of fat-free packaged foods. They often contain "mystery chemicals," don't taste that great, and destroy any sense of portion control, which is necessary for a lifetime of keeping off extra weight.

6. **RESTAURANT REMINDERS:**

   If you eat in a restaurant daily, pretend you're eating at home and follow the seven habits in the book.

   a) If lunch can be a choice of eating in a restaurant daily or brown-bagging it, take a minute to pack your own lunch. (If wearing my financial planner hat, I would say, "You'll save money.") If you keep on hand the things you like for lunch, then making your own lunch in the morning (or the night before) will take only a minute. I'm a night person, so it was easier for me to make a bag lunch for the next day before I hit the hay each night. I invested in a thermal lunch sack and bought things like precut and peeled carrots to have ready to go in the fridge. Save the lunch out for your friend's birthday or a client meeting.

   b) If social dinners out occur more nights per week than not, eat what you like; just be sure to ask for the to-go box right away— or ask the waiter to pack half the meal in a box before it's served, or share a meal with a husband or friend. Restaurant meals are supersized and it's easy to eat the whole thing. Don't do it. You will be so happy to see that doggie bag of lasagna in the fridge the next day when you open the door and ask yourself, "What's for lunch?"

7. **TAKE TIME FOR YOURSELF:**

   a) Avoid negative, defeatist self-talk. Here are some examples: "I'm so fat now." "I've just put back 10 of the 20 pounds I lost, so why try?" "I've always been overweight, so I guess I'm just genetically destined to be fat."

   b) Avoid rationalization traps:

   "I didn't eat breakfast or lunch, so I'm entitled to eat a huge dinner today."

   "My spouse loves me as I am."

   "I'm not into fashion anyway."

   "This chocolate cake is so special, I'll eat three pieces now and then I won't have dessert for a week to make up for it."

"I'm pregnant, so it doesn't matter if I gain a little extra weight."

"I'll go on a diet when I get back from vacation."

c) It might be hard to catch yourself in negative self-talk, because sometimes it's such a habit that we don't even know we are doing it. The same is true of rationalizations. The answer is to talk out loud not just to yourself. Share your thoughts about yourself with a spouse or trusted friend. Those who love you want to help you out of the negativity because they love you. Saying something out loud gets it out of your system and lets you see how such thoughts are usually without meaning or value. Revisit the reflections in this book and/or use another contemplative or motivational book of choice and read a paragraph or two every day. Visit a therapist, a pastor or rabbi, a dietitian. Personal time and centering are the keys to weight loss and lifetime weight maintenance.

QUICK TIPS FOR THE LONG TERM

- If you feel like your clothes are getting a bit tight and you are gaining weight, eat a packaged dinner two or three nights a week until the button on your jeans is no longer tight. Packaged dinners have a controlled amount of food. This will help get you back on track as to how much food to eat per meal. The packaged dinner doesn't have to be low-fat, but there are many very tasty low-fat ones on the market.

- Try the low-fat version of whatever it is you are buying: yogurt, cheese, milk, jam, peanut butter, lunch meat, and the like. If you don't mind the low-fat version, stick with it. Otherwise, eat the one you like. If you don't like a low-fat yogurt, for example, it will just sit in the refrigerator until the cows make more. You won't eat any yogurt at all, and you will have wasted money because it will just rot in the refrigerator. I found this out firsthand. I eat full-fat yogurt, a food with many health properties. Experts say it can actually help in the weight-loss process. Just be careful of the added sugars in flavored yogurt. I eat a lot of plain yogurt flavored with a bit of honey sometimes and fresh fruit. On the other hand, I can't tell the difference between full- and low-fat Swiss cheese, so I choose the low-fat version.

• When in a restaurant, ask the waiter to put a part, not necessarily half if you are just beginning to lose weight, of the entrée in a to-go box before the entrée is served to you. You will be surprised to find that you don't miss it. Never say when the full entrée is served, "I'm going to take half of this home." I never have the willpower to do that.

• If there is a food you especially love and know you can't leave alone, and you will possibly eat the whole thing in one sitting, don't buy it except on special occasions. *Never* having said food will only cause binging. For example, I love Nutella. No matter how large the jar, I can always finish it after dinner. There are about four thousand calories in a 20-ounce jar of Nutella. It also helps to have a husband who glares at me when I grin in the Nutella aisle of the grocery store and start to reach for a jar of it. Maybe your binge food is ice cream or potato chips (two of the most common I hear about). Don't buy potato chips or ice cream. Your family probably doesn't need it either. However, if you must buy potato chips and ice cream, for example, for other family members, buy single servings and play a family game of keeping count of the servings and who eats them. This will help everyone in the family maintain weight without dieting or feeling deprived just because you want to lose weight right now.

• If you love wine with dinner, try making wine spritzers, a mix of wine and sparkling water. This will give the taste of wine, a bit of a buzz, and a feeling of fullness without so many calories. Also, the wine spritzer will not increase your appetite in the same way as the straight glass of wine. Why make portion control harder for yourself than it needs to be? If you usually have two or more glasses of wine with dinner, try cutting back to just one glass and eventually to spritzers. Relish the special glass or two of wine on the occasional evening when you dine out.

• I'm always on a budget and concerned about what I spend. I always try the store-name brand of food first, for example. However, when it comes to your waistline, it's sometimes better to spend a few extra pennies than to gain a few extra pounds. For example, I go to Marie Callender's and see that whole pies are on sale for $7.95. Perhaps one slice of the pie of my choice to-go is $3.95. You know where I'm headed with this one. I have to buy the whole pie to save money, right? Don't do it. Buy the slice. In terms of real dollars spent, you have actually just saved four dollars.

- *Be sure that what you eat is very satisfying.* Don't waste calories on fattening things you don't care about; don't eat something just because it's there. On the other end, don't try to live on carrots and celery unless you're the Easter Bunny, because in the end you will just head for the chocolate from feelings of deprivation. How about if you want a ham sandwich with potato chips? Use whole wheat bread instead of white bread or a bagel. Have a small side of carrot sticks instead of potato chips. Use a little mustard on the bread instead of mayonnaise. Two ounces of potato chips (can we ever really eat only one ounce?) have 310 calories; eight carrot sticks have 35 calories. A plain white small bagel has 216 calories; two slices of whole wheat bread have 160 calories. A serving of mayonnaise has 90 calories, while a serving of mustard has three calories. By making three "better" choices, you just saved 418 calories. Eating 500 calories less per day equals 3,500 calories less per week, which equals about one pound of weight loss. Just think of how many pounds per year could be lost and from then on maintained in this way. Small changes to a ham sandwich that are barely noticeable can result in a double-digit number of pounds lost per year, and can help maintain weight loss over a lifetime.

- *Do a few extra pounds really matter?* In the beginning, no; over a lifetime, yes. In the convent, our bodies were hidden behind mounds of black serge. A collared loose cape covered the waistline. The skirt was long and slimming. When I put on the postulant's habit on my first day in the convent, I felt 50 pounds lighter already. As you begin the Convent Diet, always consider wearing a column of color, following the dress guidelines in Holy Habit #1—Visualization: You're Thin Until You're Thin"—and don't focus on pounds, to help you stick with it. After reaching a weight goal, *be vigilant*, especially during times of life-changing events, such as marriage, pregnancy, or aging, with its inertia due to arthritis or medication. Gain just two pounds a year starting at age 20, and by age 70 the 50 pounds lost will have reappeared like magic. *Be vigilant.* The scale is your friend.

- Avoid the engineered chemical food discussed in Holy Habit #6, Opt Out of Diet Food. Avoid the latest kooky fad diet. Follow the Convent Diet by eating balanced, nutritious, and tasty food—just not too much.

- Leave a bite behind on your plate at the end of each meal. Do not join "the clean plate club"—or resign from it if you are already a member.

- There is no such thing as eating the wrong thing, unless, of course, you have certain medical conditions or food allergies, but there *is* such a thing as eating too much of the right things. Too much of anything is the wrong thing. Just because the label says "low-fat" doesn't mean you should eat a ton of it. Eat less, one bite at a time.

STRIP AWAY SUPERFICIAL REASONS FOR LOSING WEIGHT... ELEVEN WRONG REASONS FOR LOSING WEIGHT

The religious habit was a wonderful cover-up. Whether you were overweight or model thin, it didn't much matter. Maybe that was a subtle lesson in removing vanity from one's life. Nothing was ever said about the habit one way or the other in this regard. We all looked forward to receiving the habit after six months as a postulant. We looked forward to becoming novices, wearing the white veil (the next step toward becoming a professed sister), and receiving the black veil.

Vanity reasons for losing weight (reasons about others, not about oneself):

1. Wear fashionable clothes
2. Catch a spouse
3. Keep a spouse
4. Make a better impression in a job interview

5. Be more popular; have more friends
6. Avoid rejection
7. Impress others with good looks
8. Pressured by parent, friend, or spouse to lose weight
9. "Keep up with the Joneses" (a friend who has lost weight)
10. Solve all self-esteem problems
11. Regard the body as a temple of God; shouldn't abuse it

While these may be the "wrong" reasons for losing weight, they may also be secondary reasons for losing weight as long as the true and primary reason for losing weight comes from inside of you. We are only human after all.

Afterword: March On

The best way to move forward is to be present in the moment. Today is a gift. Do the best you can today and know that yesterday must be forgotten, as it no longer exists, and tomorrow will be a new day and has not yet arrived.

- Give yourself permission to be imperfect. Do you want to fail at being perfect, or do you want results?
- Being thin tomorrow is the result of a series of focused todays. As the saying goes, today is the first day of the rest of your life. All past failures just don't count.
- While you don't have to enter a convent to follow the Convent Diet, it pays to follow the habits of the convent:

    1. Habits must be positive to be sustainable; there are no "thou shalt nots."
    2. Habits must come from the inside out; you must own them.
    3. Habits require repetition and discipline; I never said it would be a piece of cake, but the ingredients are all here.

- Guilt is not allowed. Forget the laundry list of negative self-talk. Love yourself first and others will love you too.

Excuses are not allowed. Weight loss and maintenance are not all-or-nothing propositions. "I blew it today, so I'll just give up tomorrow and for the rest of my life." Blowing it one day leaves 364 days to carry on this year, and more again the next year and the year after that.

Glossary

Note: The following terms are based on my personal experience as they were used by the Sisters of the Blessed Virgin Mary (BVM) congregation.

Ablutions: In formal usage, the washing of one's body or part of it, as in a religious rite, as in "performing morning ablutions." Informally, one's normal bodily cleansing routine.

Aggiornamento: The term became commonly used by Catholics under Pope John XXIII, and it has two distinct meanings: an internal spiritual renewal, and an external adaptation of the Church's laws and institutions to the times. Colloquially speaking, it represented the opening of the doors and windows of an old, stuffy Catholic Church to let in the new and fresh air.

Alcove: A section of a dorm room with white curtains that gave a sister privacy. Many dorm rooms accommodated eight alcoves; turret rooms, maybe ten. Each alcove contained a twin bed and a four-drawer chest referred to as a commode.

Basin: A white bowl, approximately 14 inches in diameter, on the top of the commode; it was filled with water at bedtime and used each morning by a novice to wash her face and brush her teeth.

Canonical year: The first of two years intended to prepare a novice for making first vows.

Commode: A small dresser in each alcove in which everyday clothes and other personal items were kept.

Duties: Each postulant and novice was given some responsibility that contributed to life at the convent; for example, helping in the kitchen or sewing room, keeping a common room clean, or assisting in the sacristy.

Franciscans: An order of religious nuns. There are several different orders of nuns called Franciscans—Franciscan Sisters of Christian Charity, Sisters of the Third Order of St. Francis, Franciscan Sisters of the Eucharist, and so on.

Habit: The outerwear of BVM sisters and those in the postulate and novitiate.

Instruction: The daily teaching session in which the novice and postulant directors met with postulants and novices to talk about elements of BVM religious life, aspects of Scripture, and prayer.

Meditation: Quiet contemplation of passages from the Scriptures and spirituality. Regular periods of time—early morning and after supper—were set aside for assembling in the chapel for this.

Motherhouse: The original building (1892) and home base for the Sisters of Charity, BVM; the site of the novitiate and postulate, offices, and some residents' quarters.

Novice: A young woman in full habit with a white veil, preparing to pronounce vows after two years of study and reflection.

Novice mistress: In the Roman Catholic Church, the mistress of novices is someone who is committed to the training of the novices and the government of the novitiate of a religious institution or order.

Novitiate: An area in the motherhouse occupied by those young sisters looking to pronounce vows.

Postlude: A closing piece of music, especially for an organ, at the end of a church service.

Postulant: A young woman in the first six months of determining if she wants to continue training as a nun.

Postulate: An area in the motherhouse occupied by those seeking membership in the community.

Priests' Kitchen: A small kitchen, separate from the large commercial kitchen, in which specialty food was prepared in small quantities for priests who came daily to say Mass, as well as for special guests.

Professed sisters: BVM sisters who have made vows of poverty, chastity, and obedience and, in the days of the habit, wore a black veil.

Refectory: The dining hall.

Retreat: Days set aside for reflection and prayer, from three to seven days; a director (often a priest) offered remarks leading to reflection.

Sacristy: An area adjacent to the chapel in which the priest presider donned vestments appropriate to the ritual; novices took care of the vestments.

Schola: Originally, a musical school attached to a monastery or church. Also known as a schola cantorum. Today, it's a group of musicians, particularly ones who specialize in liturgical music. While all professed sisters, novices, and postulants sang during church services, the schola was a select group of singers who sang the more difficult and specialty parts.

Scholastic: A young woman who had made first vows and was completing her college degree.

Scholasticate: A residence for newly professed sisters to live in while completing college courses. The scholasticate in Chicago was across the street from Mundelein College, from which many scholastics received their degrees, and which was owned by the Sisters of Charity, BVM. After the 1960s, the scholasticate was renamed Wright Hall, after one of the presidents of the congregation, and became a multigenerational residence for sisters in Chicago.

Set: A group of young women who entered the community on the same date; as in, "There are 45 sisters in my set."

Trappistines: Our Lady of Mississippi Abbey is home to 15 to 20 nuns of the Order of Cistercians of the Strict Observance, more commonly known as Trappistines. The order was founded in 1098 at Citeaux, France (about 100 miles southeast of Paris), and is now composed of monks and nuns who live in more than 20 monasteries throughout the world. The referenced Trappistine Sisters in Dubuque is a cloistered order of nuns specializing in the making of delicious chocolate candy and caramels. This particular abbey, dedicated to our Blessed Mother, was founded in 1964 in Wrentham, Massachusetts. Cloistered sisters are religious women who have dedicated their lives to prayer and contemplation. Active orders work in the missions, whether as teachers or nurses or, in modern times, in other professions, helping others.

Vatican II: The Second Vatican Council, fully the Second Ecumenical Council of the Vatican, addressed relations between the Catholic Church and the modern world. 50 years ago, Pope John XXIII launched a revolution in the Catholic Church. When he announced the creation of the Second Vatican Council in January 1959, it shocked the world. There hadn't been an ecumenical council—an assembly of Roman Catholic religious leaders meant to settle doctrinal issues—in nearly 100 years. The Second Vatican Council opened on October 11, 1962, with the goal of bringing the church into the modern world. Catholics could now hear the Mass in their local language. Laypeople could take leadership roles in the church. And the church opened conversations with other faiths. For American nuns, Vatican II brought freedoms and controversies that are still playing out today.

Vesper: An evening song. It also refers to evening prayers, and then it's usually plural. Whether it's a church service or a jazz band at sunset, if it's in the evening, it's a vesper.

Vows: Poverty, chastity, and obedience. Temporary vows were made when leaving the novitiate; final vows were made after five years.

Acknowledgments

M y dear husband, John Celentano: someone who believes in me and supports my ventures and for whom the last of my "reflections" is written.

Sister Mary Alma Sullivan, BVM: In the beginning, she was my English and journalism teacher, nurturing, inspiring, and guiding. Now we laugh and share as she continues to nurture, inspire, and guide. Mary Alma has been my muse, always thinking a step ahead...asking, "What's the next idea?" while making sure the i's were dotted and the t's crossed in the present.

Sister Mira Mosle, BVM: Without Mira's initial interest and ongoing encouragement, I don't think this book would have ever been written. We have been friends since entrance day in 1965. Mira's wisdom, sound judgment, editorial skills, and personal investment in my writing kept me on a straight path, helping me avoid the tangles in the road.

Sister Teri Hadro, BVM: In our high school, Teri was the school newspaper's editor in chief, while I was on the journalism staff, led by Sister Mary Alma. Teri entered the community with me and now, as president of the congregation, has supported and inspired me at every turn as I worked on this book.

I am grateful for the love and support of all of the Sisters of Charity, BVM, who have been part of my life's journey and have supported me in many ways, including those on the leadership team and those in the archives department, such as Jennifer Head, archivist; Anita Therese Hayes, BVM; Kathy Day; their assistants; and I am grateful for each sister, whether known to me for many years or a brand-new acquaintance, who has shared her friendship and stories, as well as the set of 1965. I especially acknowledge Sister Marguerite Yezek, BVM, my first creative writing teacher, who encouraged me then and now, and Sister Marjorie Heidkamp, BVM, for her significant contribution to the book title and other book ideas.

Millie Chen, who led me into the world of social media, has shared her creativity and supported me as I learned from her how to move in this new world. Hers was the loving gift of herself and her talent; she is like the daughter I never had.

Cindy To, always available as needed, was a true jack of all trades in her assistance regarding suggestions, technology, and artwork. She worked with the generosity and kindness of a friend.

Joyce Berenson, registered dietitian and nutritionist, believed in the book idea from the beginning, was quick with suggestions when asked, and provided the substantive foreword that is a major contribution to this book.

Richard Klein, PhD, whose psychiatric practice includes working with overweight people, finds my Seven Holy Habits psychologically sound and has endorsed this book, which is deeply appreciated.

Thank you to all of those on the book publishing team, including publisher Anthony Ziccardi, Billie Brownell, Madeline Sturgeon, Devon Brown, and especially Debra Englander.

Thank you to Rachel Shuster, for her brilliant organizational ideas and detailed editing.

Thank you to Steve Harrison and the team at Bradley Communications.

For their help, support, and best wishes I would like to thank my brother David Reid; Sister Marcia Allen, CSJ; Carol McNamara; Karen Reuter; Beverly Reggie; Marian Silverman; Ellen Mangan Turzynski; and Eileen Jack Drake.

Thank you to everyone who contributed to this book and/or helped me along the writing way.

About the Author

Mary Lou Reid entered the convent as a girl of eighteen. While there she lost fifty pounds and has kept the weight off for fifty years. Here she shares her lifelong lessons learned in the convent that led to losing and keeping off the fifty pounds. After leaving the convent Mary Lou headed to New York where she worked in the arts and media business. She attended NYU business school and then relocated to Los Angeles where she completed her education in finance. Mary Lou has worked as a Certified Financial Planner for the past thirty years. She has given many seminars, written articles, and has appeared as a financial expert on TV.